My first contact with the Hunters' ministry was through a postoperative patient who presented me with a gift of their book, *Handbook for Healing*. As I read about the multitude of diseases that could be healed through ministering, I said, "Perhaps I didn't have to go to medical school." But after I saw a videotape from Charles and Frances Hunter's "Doctors' Panel" collection, I changed my attitude. It confirmed the truth that the power of the Word was healing people and that this awesome book was based on biblical principles, the same ones Jesus used. What a blessing to witness people being healed and to be used as a vessel for the Lord.

—*Dr. Phillip Goldfedder, M.D.*

How to Heal the Sick and *Handbook for Healing* are two books that every believer should read. They teach us in such a simple way how to heal the sick so that every believer can understand how easy it is to minister healing.

—*Pastor Robb Thompson*
Family Harvest Church
Tinley Park, Illinois

Charles and Frances explain the practical steps to getting the sick healed. They make it easy to understand and inspiring to do the works of Jesus.

—*Pastor Billy Joe Daugherty*
Victory Christian Center
Tulsa, Oklahoma

God's Word tells us, *"My people* [perish] *for lack of knowledge"* (Hos. 4:6). One hundred and seventy-nine doctors put their knowledge together to help Charles and Frances write an awesome book entitled *Handbook for Healing.* They have revised it and updated it so it is a volume of unlimited knowledge for you to be successful in ministering healing to the sick.

—*Mike Floyd*
Author, *Supernatural Business*

Handbook for Healing is a book that one hundred and seventy-nine doctors and chiropractors helped Charles and Frances Hunter to write. It makes it easy for anyone to lay hands on the sick and see them recover. Every Christian should carry this book around at all times.

—*Rev. Karl Strader*
Senior Pastor, Carpenter's Home Church
Lakeland, Florida

Handbook for Healing is a must because we can't all remember what we learn about how to heal the sick. This is just a gentle reminder because it gives you a concordance in the back that tells you how to minister and what to do for every disease. It is a must for every believer.

—*Curt Frankhauser*
Assistant Pastor, First Assembly of God
Fargo, North Dakota

Handbook
for
HEALING

Revised Edition

Charles ❤ Frances
Hunter

山
WHITAKER
HOUSE

HANDBOOK FOR HEALING
Revised Edition

Charles and Frances Hunter
Hunter Ministries
P.O. Box 5600
Kingwood, TX 77325-5600
www.cfhunter.org
e-mail: wec@cfhunter.org

ISBN: 0-88368-705-4
Printed in the United States of America
© 1987, 2001 by Charles and Frances Hunter

Whitaker House
30 Hunt Valley Circle
New Kensington, PA 15068
www.whitakerhouse.com

Library of Congress Cataloging-in-Publication Data
Hunter, Charles, 1920–
Handbook for healing / by Charles and Frances Hunter.
p.   cm.
ISBN 0-88368-705-4 (pbk. : alk. paper)
1. Spiritual healing.   I. Hunter, Frances Gardner, 1916–   II. Title.
BT732.5 .H77 2001
234'.131—dc21
2001004053

4 5 6 7 8 9 10 11 12 13 14 **W** 12 11 10 09 08 07 06 05 04

Contents

Foreword

This book was birthed out of a need for additional information to help people minister healing more successfully after they had read the book, *How to Heal the Sick,* and studied the video and audio tapes by the same name. When people got out in the "field" to practice, it was difficult to remember all the things they had learned in a short period of time, so they needed a quick refresher course.

An urging of the Spirit inspired us to write a book reemphasizing some of the things we had said as well as adding new information. We knew it should be in the form of a handbook, with diseases listed alphabetically for quick reference, rather than another book on healing.

To all of you who read this and put it into effect, our sincere thanks with a grateful heart because you

have caught the vision of what Jesus is saying to the
body of Christ today.

——CHARLES AND FRANCES HUNTER

Note: This book is subject to change as God gives us new understanding and new knowledge. This is not a book of proven
science, but merely a suggestion of how to define and minister to various health problems both mental and physical.

Thank You
to the Medical Profession

The following doctors have contributed through their attendance and medical knowledge at our doctors' panels. Much of what we have learned has come from what they so unselfishly shared.

Other doctors have been on panels or with us at Healing Explosions whom we may have missed, and others will be with us in the future. We sincerely appreciate the credibility they add and the immense help to us and the healing teams.

Dr. Charles P. Adamo, B.A., Doctor of Chiropractic
Dr. Robert Aikman, M.D., C.M., Gynecology
Dr. Alexander, Doctor of Chiropractic
Dr. Peter Alderson, Doctor of Chiropractic
Dr. Larry Barge, M.D.

Dr. Raj Beliram, M.Sc. P.H.D., Pathology

Dr. David Bigby, M.D., Psychiatry

Dr. Paul Boegel, D.D.S., Peridontist

Dr. Dale C. Clark, Doctor of Chiropractic

Dr. Thomas Davis, M.D., Psychiatry

Dr. Michael Dunn, M.D., Surgeon

Dr. Burton Dupuy, Optometrist

Dr. Norman L. Dykes, M.D., Internal Medicine

Dr. H. Bruce Ewart, Ph.D., Counselor

Dr. W. Douglas Fowler, Jr., M.D., Surgeon

Dr. Ralph Gardner, Doctor of Chiropractic

Dr. Thomas Gorman, M.D., Ophthamology

Dr. Wayne Graves, Doctor of Osteopathy

Dr. Charles Guessner, D.D.S.

Dr. Steve Gyland, M.D., Pediatrics

Dr. Gerald Hall, Doctor of Chiropractic

Dr. David Hartz, M.D., General Practice

Dr. Richard Henderson, M.D., Psychiatrist

Dr. E.T. Hesse, Jr., Doctor of Chiropractor

Dr. Roger Hill, Optometrist

Dr. Randy Horton, Doctor of Osteopathy

Dr. Jeff Howard, Doctor of Chiropractic

Dr. Carol Hunt, M.D., Anesthesia

Dr. Paul Jacobs, D.D.S.

Dr. Richard Janson, M.D., Ophthamology

Dr. Richard Jantzen, M.D.

Dr. Joy M. Johnson, M.D., Radiology

Dr. Frank Keller, M.D., Preventative Medicine

Dr. Ben Kitchings, M.D.

Dr. Alice Lane, Homeopathy/Nutrition

Dr. Roy LeRoy, Doctor of Chiropractic

Dr. Jonathan Lewis, M.D., F.A.C.S., Orthopedic Surgeon

Dr. Caroline Love, M.D., Internal Medicine

Dr. Donald Loveleth, M.D.

Dr. Joseph C. Mantheis, Doctor of Chiropractic

Dr. Marilyn Maxwell, M.D., Internist

Dr. John H. McDonald, M.D., Doctor of Chiropractic

Dr. Alex Millhouse, Doctor of Chiropractic

Dr. Patrick E. Murray, Doctor of Chiropractic

Dr. Beulah Nichols, Ph.D.

Dr. Doran L. Nicholson, Doctor of Chiropractic

Dr. Larry Norville, M.D., Podiatrist

Dr. Larry Norup, M.D., Podiatrist

Dr. Thomas A. Owen, Doctor of Chiropractic

Dr. Suzanne M. Peoples, M.D.

Dr. Madelyn Permutt, Doctor of Chiropractic

Dr. Robert C. Pfeiler, M.D., Psychiatrist

Dr. Harrison Prater, Doctor of Chiropractic

Dr. Curt Priest, M.D., Emergency Medicine

Dr. James Price, D.D.S.

Dr. Frank Pushtarina, Doctor of Chiropratic

Dr. Daniel Reierson, Doctor of Chiropractic

Dr. Kenneth Romanoff, D.D.S.

Dr. R.J. Rozich, Doctor of Chiropractic

Dr. Ozzie Sailor, M.D., Surgeon

Dr. Steven G. Seifert, Doctor of Chiropractic

Dr. Robert Shiffman, Doctor of Chiropractic
Dr. Jeff Sitron, Doctor of Chiropractic
Dr. James R. Slusher, Doctor of Chiropractic
Dr. Gerald W. Spencer, D.D.S., Orthodontics
Dr. Charles Stanback, M.D., Family Practice
Dr. Thomas Stanley, M.D., Pediatrician
Dr. Dan Strader, Nutritionist
Dr. Anthony Sunseri, D.D.S.
Dr. Mary Ruth Swope, Nutritionist
Dr. Terry Terrell, D.D.S., Periodondist
Dr. David Thompson, Doctor of Chiropractic
Dr. Michael Vanaria, Doctor of Chiropractic
Dr. Larry White, Doctor of Chiropractic
Dr. Joel Wise, Doctor of Chiropractic
Dr. James Wyllie, Doctor of Chiropractic
Gene Clark, R.N.
Georgia Cohen, R.N.
Marilyn Howe, R.N.
Ella Jansen, R.N.
Betty Mills, R.N.
Yvonne Moffit, R.N.
Bobby Smith, R.N.
Ouida Walsh, R.N.

Chapter One

The Sovereignty of God

by Frances

*Hallelujah! I want to express publicly before his people my
heartfelt thanks to God for his mighty miracles. All who
are thankful should ponder them with me. For his miracles
demonstrate his honor, majesty, and eternal goodness.*
—Psalm 111:1–3 TLB

Praise God, we serve a God of miracles—a God
who wants us to walk in the supernatural and
to see miracles happen just like they did when
Jesus walked on this earth—just like His disciples
did.

"Jesus Christ is the same yesterday, today, and forever"
(Hebrews 13:8 TLB).

Praise God, we serve an unchanging God. If we truly believe with our entire being that Jesus is the same yesterday, today, and forever, then we will have to believe that He is going to be doing the same miracles today that He did yesterday and that He is going to be doing tomorrow. Only this time, He is going to be doing them by using the people He lives in and through.

Jesus said,

> *In solemn truth I tell you, anyone believing in me shall do the same miracles I have done, and even greater ones, because I am going to be with the Father. You can ask him for anything, using my name, and I will do it, for this will bring praise to the Father because of what I, the Son, will do for you. Yes, ask anything, using my name, and I will do it!*
>
> (John 14:12–14 TLB)

If Jesus said it, it has to be true! The believers are going to do exactly the same things He did, and even greater things! Not because of our own righteousness or power, but just because Jesus said we would.

We often use the latter part of that Scripture as a regular prayer Scripture, but we need to realize the conditions under which we can ask Him for anything: we must be out doing the miracles that He said we would do!

We praise God for every miracle we see, whether it is accomplished in an airport, a television station, a grocery store, an office, a service station, or a church. We love to tell people about the miracles that happen, because their faith is ignited for miracles to happen to them and through them! God not only wants us to be on the receiving end of miracles, but He also wants us to be on the performing end.

In Hosea 4:6, it says, *"My people are destroyed for lack of knowledge"* (NKJV).

But today, people are hungry for knowledge and are aggressively seeking it so that they can actually do the miracles and walk in the supernatural just like Jesus said we would.

At our Healing Explosions, we saw evidence over and over again of how people who are trained to heal the sick are shocked that they, too, can operate in the supernatural. They look at their hands and say, "I didn't believe God could use me this way!"

Today is the hour of the believer, when God is calling all believers to begin to do the things He wants us to do. Christianity is not a religion of going to church on Sunday morning, getting pumped full of Scripture and inspiring sermons, and then sitting on them for a week until we go back to church and listen again.

Christianity is a way of life! It is saying and doing the same things Jesus did, and walking in the same steps He did! Paul preached so powerfully,

> *I have been crucified with Christ; it is no longer I who live, but Christ lives* **in** *me; and the life which I now live in the flesh I live by faith in the Son of God, who loved me and gave Himself for me.*
> (Galatians 2:20 NKJV, emphasis added)

We need to understand with our hearts and not with our minds that Jesus Christ is actually living inside of us, wanting to manifest Himself to the world through us!

This is truly the hour of the believer, when God is speaking to our hearts and telling us to get off of the padded, comfortable pews and get into the arena where we can begin to do the work He has called us to do.

The five-fold ministry is "*for the equipping of the saints for the work of ministry, for the edifying of the body of Christ*" (Ephesians 4:12 NKJV). The five-fold ministry of the apostle, the prophet, the evangelist, the pastor, and the teacher is for teaching, training, maturing, and educating, the body of Christ in how to perform the work Jesus said we would do. Too long we have felt that the five-fold ministry was to do all the work and let the saints rest. No more; this is the hour of power, and this is the hour of action when the sleeping giant is coming into its own.

No longer are we to be a weak, spineless church without power and miracles, but a powerful church walking in the supernatural at every service and every hour of every day.

Charles and I have just gone through our Bibles and circled everything in the book of Acts that has to do with the supernatural. Almost everything is circled! Why? Because that early church is the prototype of what the church should be today.

Believers should be (and many are) going out and doing miracles in their everyday lives.

During a photography session the other day, we were asked to pose. We both answered the same way at the same time: "Let us talk and tell you what we do, and then when you get the right expression, take the picture!"

Because we love to talk about Jesus and what He is doing in the world today, we began to share some of the miracles that happened during our Healing Explosions and happen in our daily lives as we walk among the people!

Time came to change the film. One of the photographers stepped out and said, "I have a problem with my neck. It hurts all the time, and I am in constant agony."

Glory! Here was an opportunity for Jesus! We said, "No problem," laid hands on her, did "the neck thing," and she was instantly healed!

The film was back in the camera, so we continued to share more miracles telling what God is doing today. Then came time for another film change.

Another person walked up and said as she wheezed, "I have terrible asthma. Can you do anything about that?"

We said, "No problem," and we bound the devil in the name of Jesus, cast out the spirit of asthma, commanded new lungs to form, and commanded the bronchial tubes to be opened along with the air sacs. Suddenly, the wheezing stopped, and she was taking deep breaths.

They were ready to shoot again. Then once again came time to change film. Another individual jumped out from the back of the studio and said, "I was in an automobile accident years ago and got a whiplash. Can you do anything about that?"

We did "the total thing," and this Jewish man was instantly healed by the power of God and the authority we have in the name of Jesus!

When we left to return to the office, Charles looked at me and said, "That was a day just like the disciples had when they were here, wasn't it?" That's the way every day should be in the life of a Christian!

The next day we went to Cleveland, Ohio, to be on a television program. When we returned home, we saw a friend in the airport whom we had not seen for several years. He was meeting his mother who happened to be on the same plane we came in on, so he introduced us, and she said, "I have a horrible fungus in my throat, and I can hardly swallow. Can you help me?"

What better place to do a miracle than in a busy airport? I laid hands on her, and her throat was instantly healed. Then she told us that she had just had a bladder operation and was in pain. Charles immediately did "the pelvic thing" (yes, right on the busy concourse of the airport) and "the leg thing," and she could not believe what had happened right in front of her eyes. Even her arthritic knee was healed. Her husband received the baptism with the Holy Spirit a few minutes later—also in the airport.

As we went to get our car, we were both praising God and thanking Him for demonstrating His honor, majesty, and eternal goodness through the miracles we had just seen and that He had done through two people who happen to believe the Word of God is true and applicable to today!

Through the Healing Explosions, we have seen many people whom we have trained step out in faith and believe that God wants to use them. Through the doctors' panels, we have learned many things that have been of tremendous help to us. We are now seeing a significant increase in the percentage of people healed by the power of God through the name of Jesus!

One of the most important things we need to remember at all times is that miracles can only be accomplished by the power of God's Holy Spirit and the name of Jesus. Jesus said, *"All authority has been given to Me in heaven and on earth"* (Matthew 28:18 NKJV).

Every bit of God's authority had been given to Him, but look what He said in Luke 10:19:

> *Behold, I give **you** the authority to trample on serpents and scorpions, and over **all** the power of the enemy, and nothing shall by any means hurt you.*
>
> (NKJV, emphasis added)

He turned right around and trusted us with the power that had been given to Him! Why? So we would not be powerless, but would have the same authority He had and would perform the same miracles He did!

We cannot accept part of the Bible and then throw the rest out! If we believe He came to save us from sin and to bring us into eternal life, then we must believe the rest—even where He tells us to go out and do the same things He did!

Jesus said it was not by His power that He did miracles, but by the power of His Father. That same Holy Spirit has been given to us with the same unlimited power so that we can accomplish what needs to be accomplished on the earth today. Let's use it and enjoy it!

There is a very fine line in teaching people that the authority and power has been given to us to use. We must make sure that we take no credit for ourselves, but that we thank God and give Him all the praise and the glory for everything that is accomplished, even though we are the vessels He uses.

We can get caught up in false humility and believe that we have no ability, and yet by the same token, we can get caught up in ego and pride and take all the credit for ourselves. We need to remember that the glory for every miracle that happens belongs to God!

He has promised us that *"all the earth shall be filled with the glory of the LORD"* (Numbers 14:21). Jesus told us in the seventeenth chapter of John that we are His glory. Why are we His glory? Because we are doing the things He told us to do. We cannot ever hope to be His glory unless we are fulfilling His commandments, so that the earth will be filled with people who are casting out devils, preaching the Gospel, speaking in tongues, ministering the baptism, and healing the sick!

We praise God for the many doctors He has sent to be on our doctors' panels in the various Healing Explosions we held. We never knew who was coming, but He always brought new experts from many fields of medicine. How we praise God that we have been joined by medical doctors, orthopedic surgeons, pediatricians, obstetricians, podiatrists, chiropractors, ophthalmologists, opticians, optometrists, dentists, orthodontists, nutritionists, gynecologists, osteopaths, pathologists, surgeons, and people from other fields of medicine.

Their great medical knowledge, combined with the spiritual knowledge God gives, has brought about many healings that might not have otherwise been accomplished. Of course, remember at all times that God is sovereign, and He can perform miracles any way He chooses. Many of these doctors have told us that their lives have been completely revolutionized by what they have learned by being a part of a doctors' panel and a Healing Explosion. How we thank God for that!

Remember that we are not doctors ourselves and therefore cannot tell someone to either stop or start taking medicine. If you tell someone to take medicine, you are practicing medicine and that is illegal unless you actually are a licensed physician. After speaking healing to a person, tell them to return to his or her doctor, because healing will stand up under an examination, an x-ray, or a blood test! All the healings God has given us have stood the test of medical examinations.

People have asked, "Why don't you go and empty the hospitals?"

Probably the best reason we can give you is this: it's not legal. When you are invited by someone in a hospital or by his family or friend, it is acceptable to minister in a hospital; but even then, you need to obey hospital regulations. Don't be over-zealous and tell that person to remove his tubes or to get up and walk—then you would be practicing medicine. That determination must be made by his physician.

Even a Spirit-filled doctor who ministers to someone who is ill could not necessarily issue such an order. Only the patient's physician can give directions regarding his patient and that patient's treatment. A licensed physician must have special permission from the hospital board to practice at that facility. To be a consultant or to "practice" in another hospital, special permission must also be obtained. Though a doctor may be licensed in one state, he does not have the right to practice medicine in another state. Just as physicians must work within rules and regulations in healing the sick, so must we as ministers of God's healing power operate within specific guidelines.

God will honor a faithful and a sincere heart, but we always need to remember that God also gives us common sense and tells us to obey the law at all times. We need to confine our healing techniques to those who want to be healed by God. Jesus healed all who came to Him; He did not heal all who were in Israel.

This book is a combination of help from many doctors, information taken from the doctors' panel tapes, and things we have learned by trying more than one thing if the first one doesn't work. It is amazing how much we have learned by just out-and-out persistence.

Charles as a CPA (certified public accountant) and I as the owner of a printing company had to make things work. We carried this same tenacity into the healing ministry—we continue until we find out how God wants something done. We haven't reached 100 percent effectiveness yet; however, we will because Jesus said so!

We have done our best to put into simple terms some of the successful ways we have learned and utilized to minister healing to the sick. However, we want to remind you again that God is sovereign; and regardless of all the things you learn, He can still do it His way!

Just when we think we have something all figured out, God moves in an entirely different way. But whichever way He does it, we give Him all the praise and all the glory! We praise God for all the healings we have seen accomplished in the name of Jesus and by the power of God's Holy Spirit, whether He does it *our* way or not!

All of these are not foolproof, because if they were, then we would be God! Jesus healed *all* who came to Him, and He said we would do the same things He did. So the day is coming when the *believers* (that means you and me) will heal them *all*. The motto of all of our teaching is, "If Charles and Frances can do it, you can do it, too!" We're working toward that day when every person we touch is totally healed by the power of God working through us!

These suggestions for healing the sick have worked remarkably well for us and many other people, and we know they will also work for you. However, if you forget some of the things, just remember that with God, *all* things are possible whether you recall all the little details or not! (See Matthew 19:26.) This book is provided only as a guide and not as a rule book. We, no doubt, will discover better, more effective ways to minister healing, and so will you. We readily accept these changes so that we can increase our effectiveness in ministering healing.

Please don't memorize, but rather rely on a general understanding and the leading of the Holy Spirit. These are only guidelines. These are things we have done, or realized from doctors' panels, and because they have resulted in healings, we pass them on to you.

This *Handbook for Healing* is intended as a quick review of the book *How to Heal the Sick,* the video and audio tapes by the same name, and the pre-explosion teaching sessions. **We do not recommend that you attempt to use what we have written in this book until you have read the book *How to Heal the Sick* or studied the video and audio tapes by the same title.** This, then, is a supplement to what you have learned and can be used as a quick reference or refresher course.

Don't get discouraged if you try everything, and nothing seems to work. As Paul said, *"Having done all, to stand"* (Ephesians 6:13 NKJV). Remember, you have laid hands on them, and the power of God has gone into them. Let God's Holy Spirit "penicillin power" have time to work.

Just the other day a man approached me asking if I remembered praying for a little baby fourteen years ago who had no skull. Only the sides of the skull were present; the top was absent, revealing just a soft mass. The parents had a helmet-like contraption on the baby's head for protection. I remembered ministering to the baby. When I laid hands on him, I "saw" nothing, and since then I had heard nothing from the parents. I would love to have seen an instant miracle where the skull bones formed immediately, but God chose not to do it that way. Having done all I knew to do, I stood!

As I recalled the incident, the man reported that within two months after I laid hands on that incomplete head, the baby had a perfect skull. Today, fourteen years later, he is a healthy, normal human being! Remember, you don't always get to see your miracles, but God records them all in heaven. Glory!

I didn't learn to walk until I tried.

I didn't learn to talk until I tried.

I didn't learn to drive a car until I tried.

I didn't learn to type until I tried and kept on trying!

I didn't learn to heal the sick the first time I tried, either.

I haven't learned how to heal *all* the sick, but I'm trying, and I'm going to keep on trying until we see 100 percent of the people we lay hands on totally healed.

The desire of my heart is to see those little children who have been attacked in their mother's womb by the devil himself—who have epilepsy, mental retardation, blindness, deafness, imperfect bodies, and other deformities—totally and completely healed by the power of God when I hand them back to their parents.

I haven't seen many such instant healings of afflicted children as yet, but I'm going to keep trying and learning all I can until manifestations of total healing become a reality not only in our lives, but in yours as well.

Jesus came to seek and to save the lost, and He used healing as a tool. He wants us to do exactly the same thing. There is nothing that will convince a sinner of the reality of Jesus faster than witnessing a miracle.

One of our healing schools in Israel was contacted by a Jewish family who needed a healing miracle. They resisted the use of Jesus' name, but finally said it could be used if the healing team felt it was absolutely necessary. The man had a back problem as a result of an accident. As the healing team ministered to him in the name of Jesus, he was completely healed.

The wife had told them she had a problem with her lungs. When the healing team asked her if they could lay hands on her, she said, "When you grew out my husband's legs and his back was healed, that blue flame that came out of your hands came right across the room into my lungs. I'm healed!"

Then the husband said, "If that is Jesus, we want to accept Him as our Messiah!" They both were saved that day! A miracle is worth a million words!

For that woman to be allowed to see blue flames shoot across a room and into her lungs was a sovereign act of God and a sign to a Jewish couple. So regardless of how much we learn about healing the sick (and we should learn as much as possible), let us never underestimate the sovereignty of God.

He can perform miracles and healings any way He wants to!

One of the most thrilling things in our ministry is to see how the believers are latching on to the idea that God actually does want all of us to lay hands on the sick, and that Jesus sent the Holy Spirit so we would all have the same power, authority, and responsibility that He had to heal the sick. Jesus lives in us and does His work through us.

You and I are living in the most exciting days in which a Christian has ever had the opportunity to live. You and I are seeing the demonstrations of the Holy Spirit that have not been seen even in the days of the disciples.

Recently we were ministering on "The Holy Ghost and Fire," when suddenly the pastor stood up and said, "I'm about to freak out!" I was so shocked when he said this because I wondered what I had said that caused his reaction. But he continued, "I hear the wind of the Spirit blowing! It's so awesome, I'm scared!" Seven hundred and fifty people who were at that meeting instantly stood up and screamed, "I hear the wind, too!"

We all want to go up on a higher level where the Holy Spirit is concerned. God wants us to believe that He is who He says He is, that He can do any-thing, and that absolutely nothing is impossible with Him. We all say it with our mouths. We all say it with our heads—"Nothing is impossible with God." But we need to get it way down deep into our hearts. When we say, "Nothing is impossible with God," we need to believe it with all of our minds, our hearts, our bodies, and our souls, and believe that Jesus can do all things through us.

Head knowledge is no good. Lip service is no good. It has to be so deep in your heart that you don't ever limit God. We're so foolish when we limit God, because if God created the universe, He can do anything. He can do anything and *everything!* And He will do it for you, *through Jesus* (Hebrews 1:2 and Colossians 1:16 NLT) and through you!

THINK ON THESE THINGS

by Madeline Permutt, D.C.

"A merry heart doeth like a medicine: but a broken spirit drieth the bones" (Proverbs 17:22). When we laugh, when we are happy, when we praise God, when we exercise, *endorphins* are released in our bodies. Endorphins relieve pain and are healing (act as "medicine") to the tissues of our body. Synthetic morphine was patterned after endorphins. God is so good! Amen!

And, of course, the contrary is true. If we are not joyful, if we do not praise God, if we don't exercise, the endorphins do not flow, and we experience pain and sickness (and *"a broken spirit drieth the bones"*).

Chapter Two

When You Touch God

by Charles

In 1969, after I totally committed my life to God, He took my spirit and soul out of my body, zoomed me into space, held me in His glorious golden light, and then returned me to my earthly body. The complete story is in our books, *Follow Me* and *Born Again, What Do You Mean?*

As I looked at my spirit out of my body before my soul went into the spirit, my body looked identical to me—size, shape, and even the face was the same. The only difference was that you could see through this spirit body as if it was carved out of a thin cloud or fog.

When God made the Bible come alive to me, it was clear that when we are born again and baptized with the Holy Spirit, our spirits are filled with God's Holy Spirit. I realized then that my spirit, the size of me, was actually and literally filled full of the Spirit of God. I also realized that when Jesus came into my life, He lived in me and filled my spirit and soul with His Spirit. Paul spoke of *"Christ in you, the hope of glory"* (Colossians 1:27), and if the Spirit of Christ is not in you, you are not a Christian. (See Romans 8:9.)

I love the way Jesus put it, and love it most in *The Living Bible:*

> *My prayer for all of them is that they will be of one heart and mind, just as you and I are, Father—that just as you are in me and I am in you, so they will be in us, and the world will believe you sent me.*
>
> (John 17:21 TLB)

When I touch your finger, I am touching God and Jesus. When I touch the top of your head or the bottom of your feet, I am touching God and Jesus in you.

By knowing this, I know that the power of God's Holy Spirit from within me is what heals the sick and sets the captives free. Jesus said, "I felt healing virtue go out of me." (See Luke 8:46.) That's the power that heals the sick.

If I went to a doctor with an infection in my body, after diagnosing it, he would possibly say, "Nurse, give him two *ccs* of penicillin, and that will kill the infectious germs." Suppose the nurse came back to the doctor holding a bottle of penicillin and the syringe needle and said, "Doctor, I don't know how to get this out of the bottle and into his body." Suppose the doctor answered, "I don't either."

Would the penicillin heal my sickness? Of course not! When our spirits are totally and completely filled with God's Holy Spirit, we still must know how to dispense this Holy Spirit "penicillin" into the bodies of the sick people to heal them. It is God's Holy Spirit power that heals, and the simple principle of healing is to dispense this power from the Spirit of God within our spirits into the bodies of the sick people.

Let's examine the way a doctor "heals" the sick. We will assume that we have caught a germ of some kind and have made an appointment to see our doctor. He examines us and gives us his diagnosis.

Then he prescribes a certain amount of penicillin or other medication and says, "That should cause you to get over this in two or three days."

You go home, and what happens? In two or three days you are well. Did the doctor heal you? No, he used his skill and knowledge and understanding to discover what was wrong, and he prescribed the proper medication for the problem. Did the nurse who injected the medicine heal you? No.

What healed you, then? The penicillin or other prescribed medication did.

Divine healing is similar in principle. The power is injected by the laying on of hands for healing, but it is the Giver of power who gets all the credit.

When we receive the baptism "with" or "in" the Holy Spirit, we have the most dynamic healing power of all within us. We are endued with the power of the Holy Spirit of the almighty God! (See Luke 24:49.) What an honor! What a privilege! What a responsibility! When this divine power is dispensed into a sick body, the power does the healing. We always give glory to God and Christ Jesus. Always, when ministering healing, do it in the name of Jesus.

You Are a "Light Switch"

If you have ever turned a light switch on or off, you're smart enough to heal the sick!

Somewhere, not too far from where you are, is a generator (a power plant) that produces electricity. A wire brings this electricity, this power, from the source to your house and up to your electric bulb. The energy flowing from the power plant to the light bulb causes the filament of the bulb to illuminate. When this happens, we say the light is "on."

Between the power plant and the light bulb is a switch or breaker. The switch is designed to break the flow of energy, the power, from its source to the destination in the light bulb. If you turn on the switch, the two ends of the wire are connected and the energy will flow through. If it is turned off, the wires are separated, and the energy cannot continue because of the gap between the power source and the light bulb.

In the same way, the Holy Spirit in you is the generator or the power plant—the source of the power. Your hands are the on and off switch, and the person needing healing is the light bulb.

Now it is entirely up to you whether you turn the light switch on or off. It is entirely your choice in healing to lay hands on the sick. Actually, the only choice you have is whether or not you will be obedient to the command of Jesus.

The power of God will do the healing, just as the electric current will light the bulb. If you want a dark room to light up, you can turn on the light switch. If you don't flip the switch, the room will stay dark. If you have an opportunity to minister healing to someone, it is the same kind of choice. You can lay hands on that person and see him recover, or you can let him remain sick.

If you have not yet received your "generator," do so right now. Ask Jesus to baptize you with the Holy Spirit. Lift your hands up to God and begin to praise Him, but not in any language you know. Start expressing sounds of love so the Holy Spirit can take whatever sounds you give Him and give you the language that will turn any ordinary individual into an extraordinary person! Let your spirit soar as it talks to God for the very first time. (See 1 Corinthians 14:2.)

Be a light switch for Jesus, but be sure you are "turned on" for Him. Jesus said, *"You are the light of the world"* (Matthew 5:14 NKJV). Let this be part of your being the light of the world.

Laying hands on the sick and healing them is one means that Jesus used to be the light of the world, to illuminate the way for the lost to find Him. He passed this earthly job on to us and gave us this healing virtue, this dynamic power, so that we could effectively carry on all of His work while we are on earth.

As you study the book *How to Heal the Sick,* you will see the explanations given as to how to dispense this power through laying on of hands, commanding, putting faith into action, casting out demons,

When You Touch God 🖤 *39*

and other ways Jesus and the disciples used to minister healing to the sick.

Jesus said that you are to lay your hands on the sick and heal them (Mark 16:18 TLB). The *New King James Version* of the same verse says that *"they will recover."*

Tens of thousands of believers who have learned through our book and video and audio tapes how to dispense the power of God's Holy Spirit in Jesus' name are seeing miracles happen daily just like Peter, James, John, Paul, and the others did in the early church.

HEALING: A LIFESTYLE

Healing is simple, easy, and uncomplicated because it is all done with God's power in the name of Jesus! Healing was a lifestyle for Jesus and for the early disciples, and it should be exactly the same today for every born-again, Spirit-filled Christian on earth.

However, since the time when the disciples lived on earth, only a few people—mostly ministers—have been gifted with what is called a healing ministry or gifts of healing. During this generation, ordinary Christians have discovered that they, too, can do what Jesus told all of us to do.

There is a big difference between the gifts of healing and simply being obedient to the commands Jesus gave us. The gifts of healing are still present in a number of Christians, but all Christians have a responsibility to obey everything Jesus told us to do. In Mark 16:18, He said that those who believe *"will lay hands on the sick, and they will recover"* (NKJV). This is a lifestyle Jesus was talking about—not a special gift, but a normal sign and wonder that would follow all believers to confirm the fact that they were telling the truth when they spoke about His miracle-working power.

Healing is not an end unto itself, but it is a God-given tool for us to use, just as Jesus and the disciples did, so that people will believe in Jesus Christ as their Savior and Lord and be born again. It is most certainly a tool that is vitally needed by Christians today. But even more important, it is probably the best tool we have been given to aid in the evangelization of souls. When individuals are healed by the power of God, it is extremely difficult for them not to believe in Jesus as their Savior!

As fanatical as we were about wanting to learn how to heal the sick, we never lost sight of the purpose of healing:

> *Jesus' disciples saw him do many other miracles besides the ones told about in this book, but these are recorded*

*so that you will believe that he is the Messiah, the Son
of God, and that believing in him you will have life.*
                    (John 20:30–31 TLB)

Jesus laid hands on the sick, and they recovered.

Jesus commanded fever to leave, and it obeyed.

Jesus spoke to diseases and evil spirits, and they
left.

But, strangely, Jesus never "prayed" for the sick.
He healed them! Paul "healed" the sick, too. (See
Acts 28:8.) A light began to shine in our hearts, and
a key of understanding opened a door of healing for
us.

Chapter Three

Falling under the Power

by Charles

We know from tens or hundreds of thousands on whom we have laid hands that the Holy Spirit does deep healing of spirits, sickness, injuries, depression, attitudes, habits, hurts, abuses, and other needs when they fall under the power of God. This is often referred to as being slain in the Spirit, resting in the Spirit, dormission, or falling under the power.

This happened to Paul on the road to Damascus when Jesus appeared to him; it happened to the squadron of soldiers and Judas when they came to capture Jesus; it happened to John on the Isle of Patmos (see Revelation), and many other people in the Bible.

We believe that the power of the Holy Spirit that brings forth this phenomenon is the same power that heals the sick. God's power will reach into the inner recesses of our very souls to do a work much greater than could be done by all the ministry in the world. That is why we lay hands on people even after their healing has been completed. We want them to receive ministry of the Holy Spirit for all their inner needs as well as physical healings.

In our own lives, Frances had every hang-up in the book concerning the baptism with the Holy Spirit, when Kathryn Kuhlman called her out of an audience and laid hands on her to go under the power. God knew the need of her life and mine, and when she came up from the floor, she did not have a single objection to the baptism with the Holy Spirit. Shortly after that, we both received the baptism. God had met the need!

After you have ministered healing, simply lay hands on the person's forehead or temples and say, "Jesus, bless him!" Make sure you have a catcher behind him as you allow the power of God to touch him and minister to him. However, if he does not fall under the power, do not be concerned.

We do not recommend anyone touching or talking with someone while he is under the power, because God is doing a work, and He doesn't need your help!

Chapter Four

The Gifts of the Spirit

by Charles

Jesus said *all* believers would lay hands on the sick and they would recover. He said *all* believers would cast out devils, speak in tongues, and handle the old serpent, the devil, and all his poisons. He said *all* believers would minister healing to the sick.

All believers, if obedient to Jesus, will do all of the above things in their daily walk with God and Jesus. However, Paul said something very positive about the gifts of the Spirit:

Now concerning spiritual gifts, brethren, I do not want you to be ignorant....There are diversities of gifts, but the same Spirit. There are differences of ministries, but

> *the same Lord. And there are diversities of activities, but it is the same God who works all in all. But the manifestation of the Spirit is given to each one for the profit of all: for to one is given the word of wisdom through the Spirit, to another the word of knowledge through the same Spirit, to another faith by the same Spirit, to another gifts of healings by the same Spirit, to another the working of miracles, to another prophecy, to another discerning of spirits, to another different kinds of tongues, to another the interpretation of tongues. But one and the same Spirit works all these things, distributing to each one individually as He wills.* (1 Corinthians 12:1, 4–11 NKJV)

All of us need to lay hands on the sick as Jesus said, but not all are necessarily qualified to operate in the gifts of the Spirit. The gifts of healing are entirely different from laying hands on the sick. It is a supernatural endowment of the power of God that is normally manifested in services where there are large audiences, and not generally as hands are being laid on people individually, although it can be.

Recently a young boy was sleeping through one of our services because he was 95 percent deaf and could hear nothing that was being said. His mother had brought him to have hands laid on him at the end of the service, but a supernatural gift of healing was present, and suddenly the boy woke up, stood up, placed his hands over his ears and said, "Let's get out of here, Mother; it's too noisy. It's hurting my ears!"

He had been supernaturally healed by the power of God without any human being ministering to him. I tested his ears at the end of the service, and even though I stood several feet behind him and whispered, he could hear every word I said! That particular gift does not operate at all times, but it is a sign and wonder and an indication of a real move of God in a service.

Two of these gifts that are mentioned and about which we want to give you a little input are two gifts that can be invaluable in healing the sick, but can also be a dangerous tool in the hands of an unseasoned Christian. They are the word of wisdom and the word of knowledge.

Our daughter Joan operates mightily in these gifts, having matured greatly in this area by opening up her spirit to hear the voice of God. Almost all of these gifts are merely the result of being able to hear God and then relaying what He said, and they are powerful if used correctly. However, not *all* have these gifts. Paul said to "one" is given this gift and "to another" is given another gift, so we will not all operate in these gifts.

Wonderful things can happen if we are operating in the Spirit and not in the flesh, but terrible things can happen if we operate in the flesh! Immature Christians have a tendency to think in terms of what they *want* to happen and not what God is actually saying, and they can step in front of God's plans. Sometimes we don't even look for what we actually *want* to happen, but something that will bring glory or praise to us.

We have heard unseasoned Christians, in their attempts to operate in the word of knowledge, say, "God just told me that you have cancer and are dying." The person to whom this word has been given will be panic stricken at the thought of having cancer.

Much harm and damage can be brought about by an immature, careless, self-seeking person, even though he is sincere, when he attempts to operate in the gifts of the Spirit.

A woman fancied herself in love with one of the singers in a group who previously traveled with us, and she told him this interesting story. "I see a spirit of death hovering over you. God told me the only way to remove it was for you to divorce your wife and marry me!"

We know this is an isolated case, but this happens often to other people. This young man was frightened and asked us if we saw a spirit of death over him. We assured him we did not, and we told him to forget what he had heard.

By Frances

The word of knowledge is invaluable in healing, because many times people do not tell or even know the truth about what is actually wrong with them. Many years ago a woman came to our service who had not spoken in years. She had been normal up until twenty years prior to her attending one of our services. I questioned her as to whether or not there had been a sickness of some kind, a high fever, or some other physical problem, and as we stood there, God said, "Twenty years ago she saw her husband murder another man. She did not want to testify against him, so she voluntarily lost her ability to speak."

That was a situation that required the word of wisdom along with the word of knowledge. I did not speak out and say, "God just told me you saw your husband murder another man. That's your problem!" That would have been foolishness.

When the service was over, I was talking to the pastor and casually asked him if he knew anything about this particular woman's past. He said, "Oh, yes, her husband was tried for murder years ago, and that is when this happened!"

I did not reveal to the pastor what God had said to me, but he certainly confirmed what I had heard.

The woman was still there, so I went over, laid hands on her, and asked God to remove from her mind anything that shouldn't be there, and instantly her speech returned.

The word of knowledge had been given to me personally. It had not been given so that I would blab to the world, because along with it God gave me wisdom to know how to use that word of knowledge.

The word of knowledge can be invaluable in almost any situation where you are dealing with another person, but it should be exercised first in your church under the leadership of your pastor who knows you and your spiritual maturity. This way you can be corrected, if necessary, to help you mature in this area. If you receive a word of knowledge such as I did, ask God what to do with it, and also make sure that it is God who said it in the first place.

Years ago when I was first saved, I was ministering in Sarasota, Florida, at a non-Pentecostal church. I knew nothing about the gifts of the Spirit, tongues, or anything else in that realm. I was praying for people at an altar, and a man walked up to me and said, "You have the gift of healing; why don't you use it?"

I didn't say a word, because I had no idea what he was talking about. He immediately turned, walked

toward the door, and disappeared. I've often wondered if it was an angel, but nevertheless, I didn't tell
anyone or do anything about it although I continued
doing the things I had been doing up to that time.
Obviously it was a word of knowledge that was genuine, because I have seen it come true, whether it
came through man or angel!

Prophecies given in the flesh but received as if
from God have led many good Christians astray.
We are to follow after the Holy Spirit rather than a
prophecy. When someone prophesies over us, we lay
it on the shelf until it comes true, and then we know
that person is a genuine prophet, but we never run
after the prophecy in an attempt to make it happen.
If it's of God, it will happen; if it's not, it won't. It's
as simple as that.

Don't be so eager that you ruin someone's life
with your fleshly words of knowledge or prophecy.
Desire to operate in the gifts, but only under controlled situations (such as your own church), until
you have matured sufficiently to be able to operate
in public meetings. Gifts or abilities of the Spirit are
to be used to accomplish what you are to do for God
at that time. These gifts are not given to all, but all
believers are to minister healing.

Those operating in the various abilities or gifts
of the Spirit should be mature, seasoned, Spirit-filled

Christians who love God and Christ Jesus with all their hearts, who put God's desires before their own desires, and who spend much time meditating in the Word of God.

If I were a baby Christian, I would spend hours and hours meditating in the Word of God, not seeking revelation knowledge, but seeking to know God and Jesus and learning to please them. I wouldn't trust my four-year-old granddaughter to drive a car, but as she continues to grow in the simple process of living, she will eventually become qualified to learn to drive. Until then, we're going to teach her the things that are suitable for her age. The same thing is true of a new Christian.

An old saying, but nevertheless a good one, is, "Don't try to run before you can walk." Little children do this, and they quickly fall and get their knees skinned! Take all the gifts of God according to your ability and maturity to operate in them. God will give you plenty of opportunities to use them to fulfill what He has called you to do.

And pastors, we'd rather have a little wildfire than no fire, because it's easier to put out wildfire than it is to kindle dead ashes!

Chapter Five

The Neck Thing

by Charles

We decided in the beginning of our ministry that God had made everything simple, and therefore we should, too. So we have entitled all the things we do in healing in a simple manner, easy to identify and easy to remember.

Sometimes it's difficult to remember where you got the first glimmer from God concerning a method of healing, and in "the neck thing" we had to go back into our memory to recall where it began and why we started doing what we're doing.

We had a guest in our home who had a pain in his toe. I "grew out" the arms and the legs, and the pain did not leave. Then I asked him what the doctor said caused the pain. We believe in doctors, and we believe if you don't get healed by divine power, you need to go to a doctor to find out what the problem is. Then we can know where and how to minister healing by God's power, and it will be easy to get healed supernaturally.

He said the chiropractor had advised him that he had a thin disc in his back; and even though it was in the lower back, the chiropractor adjusted his neck The pain had left, but it subsequently returned.

I put my two hands on his neck, placing my fingers on his upper spinal column. *"Those who believe…will lay hands on the sick"* (Mark 16:18 NKJV). At the same time, I did not realize where the other parts of my hands actually were resting. Later I discovered that the palms of my hands were on the carotid artery, which is the main artery on both sides of the neck, through which blood is pumped into the brain. Therefore, this is also applying the power of God to any part of the brain that might need attention. The palms were also on the nerves that go from the brain down the front of the body.

This automatically makes your thumbs fall right on the temporomandibular joint, which is where we have problems with what is better knows as "TMJ." You are laying hands (thumbs) on the strongest muscle of the body. Was it accidental that God made our hands so that when we placed them in the right position we would be "laying hands" on three vital parts of the body at one time? Or did He plan it so that when we started probing into how to heal the sick the supernatural way, we would discover what He knew all along?

Then, with my hands gently in place as described above, I asked the man to slowly turn his head to the left and then the right, then backward and forward. While I was doing what we later called "the neck thing" (TNT), I commanded all the muscles, ligaments, tendons, and vertebrae to go into place and the thin disc to be healed in the name of Jesus.

Then he himself rotated his head and shouted, "The pain is gone!"

We did this for four years and also discovered the results were phenomenal for headaches as well. Then one day Dr. Roy J. LeRoy, a well-known chiropractor, told us what we were actually doing and why the results were so tremendous.

We have seen outstanding healings through "the neck thing," not only in our ministry, but through the tens or hundreds of thousands whom we have taught this natural—supernatural application of God's healing power.

Almost 100 percent of neck problems, headaches, nerve deafness, arthritis in the neck, fractured vertebrae, deteriorated, herniated, or disintegrated discs, even broken necks, and TMJ have been healed by this application of God's healing power.

You will discover that large percentages of health problems will be healed through the basic healing application of "the total thing" (TTT), growing out arms and legs, "the neck thing" (TNT), and "the pelvic thing" (TPT). This not only affects the spinal system, but it also affects internal parts because nerves make muscles work properly.

Chapter Six

The Pelvic Thing

by Frances

God will give you "witty inventions" and ideas beyond your ability and capability if you will be sensitive to the Holy Spirit and move when He moves!

At a service in Jacksonville, Florida, a man came up who had "duck" feet. I certainly didn't know what to pray, except to command his feet to turn inward instead of outward, when a thought filtered into my mind. It was a real "flash" thought, but I knew that God had said something to me, and it seemed to me that He was indicating it had something to do with the spine.

A chiropractor was with us, so I asked him if there was a problem in the spine that caused this to happen and make the man's feet turn out.

He replied, "His pelvic bones are turned out and need to be turned inward." In the natural or chiropractic world, this would be difficult or impossible to do; but in God's kingdom and in the supernatural world, this is easy to do.

I placed my hands on the top of his pelvic bones and commanded the pelvis to rotate in until the feet were normal. I was probably the most surprised person there when I noticed the entire pelvic area began to turn from side to side.

I wasn't doing it!

He wasn't doing it!

It had to be the power of God!

Just as quickly as the rotating had started, it stopped, and the man fell under the power of God. When he stood up again, his feet were no longer in a "duck" position, but were perfectly straight!

Once again, God had opened a natural—supernatural channel for us to learn more about healing.

It didn't take us long to figure out that if rotating in with the power of God would correct "duck" feet, then surely rotating out would correct people with pigeon toes! We tried it, and it worked. We have seen many people since that time healed of feet that turn in!

We discussed this with many doctors on our doctors' panels, and they all agreed it could be invaluable in many other diseases as well. Because of the involvement of the entire pelvic area, many female problems are healed through this simple laying on of hands. We have had hundreds of women healed of PMS (premenstrual syndrome) by this simple act of commanding the female organs to go into place while the pelvis is rotating.

Many problems in the lower lumbar area (the lower five vertebrae) and the sacrum are healed through this method. Command the vertebrae to be adjusted properly. Often a frozen or dislocated sacrum is restored to its right position by doing "the pelvic thing."

Prostate problems can be healed this way by commanding the prostate to become normal.

Colon problems are healed by commanding nerves controlling the colon to become normal.

Actually, many times, any organ or part of the body that lies between the waistline and the hips can be healed by this simple act.

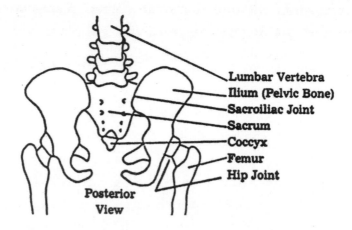

Lumbar Vertebra
Ilium (Pelvic Bone)
Sacroiliac Joint
Sacrum
Coccyx
Femur
Hip Joint

Posterior
View

The Pelvic Thing: The sacroiliac can assume many different positions. Sometimes the ilium (pelvic bone) rotates on the sacrum and causes one leg to appear short; or it can go out of position, and the legs will appear to have even lengths and still the spine is crooked (scoliosis). The sacrum can tilt forward and cause lordosis (swayback) or backward and cause a straight or "military" back. In all these examples, do the pelvic thing and command the sacrum to move into the correct position.

It never hurts to look at a picture of the human body so you will know where certain parts are located. The pelvic bones are sometimes called the hip bones. They are the flat bones that make up your skeletal structure for the hip and pelvis area. If you will run your hands down your side in the area of your waist, you will discover the tops of the bones lie right in that area, and that is where you place your fingers.

When you begin to make commands, if that portion of the body needs adjusting, the pelvis will rotate or move in one direction or the other. If nothing is needed, nothing will happen and it will not move.

Many times one side will be higher than the other, so command the high side to lower and the low side to come up. It's fabulous what the power of God can and will do!

Don't underestimate the value of this simple healing process. It is incredible what happens!

THE SCIATICA OR THE SCIATIC NERVE

Did you ever have a pain shoot down your entire leg, and you felt as if your leg was going to buckle under you? You were probably a victim of sciatica, a painful situation generally caused by a pinched nerve. This is usually caused when a disc wears thin on one side. When that happens, the spine tips on the side where the thinning disc has occurred, and this causes the body to put pressure on the sciatic nerve. This pressure then causes pain to shoot down the leg. Normally this happens only on one side or the other, depending on where the thinning has occurred. It can also be caused by a strained back, but normally it comes from a nerve that has been pinched.

This is one of the most painful of back problems, but one of the easiest to heal. It is very easy to find the exact spot once you learn where to place two fingers, because the area is always very painful and sensitive to touch. Once you discover how to locate the junction of the pelvic bone and the sacrum, lay two fingers on the area of the back (on the side where the problem is) and command the spirit of sciatica to come out in the name of Jesus. Have the person bend over. It is when the person bends over and puts his or her faith into action that the healing actually occurs.

In almost all cases, the minute he bends over and put his faith into action after you touched that sacroiliac joint, the pressure will be relieved and the person will be healed. If you will look at the diagram on page 60, you will see exactly where the sacroiliac joint is located, and it's very easy to learn exactly where to put your fingers on one side or the other. If you can imagine one of the discs being thin and the spine bending one way or the other, you will see why there will be a "pinch" in that area.

Recently an administrator of a church came to me when a service was over and said, "I can hardly walk. This pain shoots down my leg to my toe, and it's killing me!" I placed my fingers on her sciatic nerve. Before I said a word, the power of God had healed her. Laughing, she said, "It's gone!"

Chapter Seven

Electrical and Chemical Frequencies

by Charles

Your body is completely made up of cells—blood cells, skin cells, brain cells, and so on—and around all of these cells there are electrical and chemical frequencies that flow and keep them operating.

Frances and I listen and learn all the time from other people. Scientists have discovered that when the electrical and chemical frequencies in a person's body are in harmony and in balance, no disease can live in that body.

This really got our attention! Jesus healed *all* who came to Him.

The statement about disease not being able to live when the frequencies are in harmony and balance intrigued us. One of the things that we believe with our heart and soul is that if the doctors can do it with medicine and skills, we can do it with the power of God. We believers become "practicing" evangelists. Doctors are called practicing physicians because they constantly practice, so I guess we can do the same thing.

Frances and I were in a meeting, and a lady came to us who stated, "I have an environmental disease. I am in pain twenty-four hours a day, and I have lost the sight in one eye. This pain is non-stop; it never ceases." She said that she had formerly been an executive secretary, but at this particular point, the function of her mind had so deteriorated from this environmental disease that she had difficulty addressing twelve Christmas cards that year.

We thought this was an excellent thing to try out on her because you cannot lose whenever you lay hands on somebody. We said, "In the name of Jesus we command the electrical and chemical frequencies in every cell in your body to be in harmony and in balance and to digest the bad cells." In chemotherapy, which is often used on cancer patients, the chemotherapy destroys or digests the good cells as well as the bad cells. But with the electrical and chemical frequencies in balance, the good cells are not harmed whatsoever.

After we made this command on this lady, she fell under the power of God. When she got up she almost screamed because she had no pain left. She was literally jumping with joy and went dancing back to her seat, when about three or four minutes later she came up screaming and saying, "I can see! I can see! I can see!" God had instantly healed her eye and taken all the pain out. We asked her to really test this for us and to contact us in two or three weeks.

Where her mind had blanked out and she couldn't even address twelve Christmas cards three weeks previously, she wrote us a four-page letter on a computer, absolutely perfect, with perfect sentence structure and every word spelled correctly. In that letter she told us what the effects of the healing were: that her mind was brought back to normal, her eyesight was normal, and there has not been any pain in her body from that day to this!

This is the same command we made on a lady who was healed of Parkinson's disease. We have seen many similar cases healed by this very simple little command.

Recently a man around sixty years of age attended a service, suffering horribly from environmental disease that had plagued him for eighteen years. He said for all of the eighteen years, he had had nothing but excruciating, continuous pain in his body. We laid hands on him and made the very simple electrical and chemical frequency command, and he instantly fell under the power of God. He was there for quite a long time. When he got up he said, "I have no pain, but I don't want to give a testimony because I took pain medicine before I came."

He came back twenty-four hours later with an awesome testimony of no pain medication of any kind, and he said he had absolutely no pain whatsoever in his body for the first time in eighteen years!

We use this particular command on many different diseases. One with which we have been seeing some good results is Chronic Fatigue Syndrome, and another is fibromyalgia. Chronic Fatigue Syndrome is something apparently new that has cropped up in the medical field, and yet it seems like a tremendous number of people have the same comment: "I'm tired all the time. I'm exhausted. I can't seem to get rested." We make exactly the same command for that as we do the environmental disease or multiple sclerosis, cancer, muscular dystrophy, or any incurable disease.

When we ask for people who have been diagnosed with fibromyalgia, or who have bad continuous pain, not in joints or bones, but in their flesh and in all areas of their bodies to come up for healing, they come quickly, sometimes five or ten at a time. When we make the electrical and chemical frequency command, nearly 100 percent are healed, and all pain leaves immediately. What an awesome instant miracle is happening with this simple command!

Remember that it is not a prayer, because Jesus never prayed for the sick. It is a command, so firmly get it fixed in your mind to say, "In the name of Jesus, we command the electrical and chemical frequencies in every cell in your body to be in harmony and in balance and to digest the bad cells. Thank You, Jesus." We ourselves make this command by laying our fingers on our foreheads every morning at our breakfast table to start the day off right, and we suggest you do the same.

One of the most important things that we have learned in healing is for people to say "thank You" as soon as the prayer or the command is completed. Many times people are so aware of the presence of God as they are being healed that they simply forget to say anything. But encourage people to constantly say, "Thank You, Jesus; thank You, Jesus; thank You, Jesus." When you say that, what you are really saying to God is, "I've got it! I've got it! I've got it!" No one can say those three words, "Thank You, Jesus," too often.

WHAT GOES WRONG IN PARKINSON'S DISEASE?

The progressive death of nerve cells in the substantia nigra, deep within the brain, leaves the nerve fibers in the movement control centers with too little dopamine, a chemical messenger. Patients develop tremors and rigidity. Why the neurons die isn't known.

There are many commands that we use over and over again on many people, and the electrical and chemical frequencies is one of them. Two nights in a row, men came up to us with Parkinson's disease who were shaking violently, as this disease often makes one do. They said the doctors had been unable to do anything for it. Frances made the command in both instances and commanded all the electrical and chemical frequencies in every cell in their bodies to be in harmony and in balance. There is nothing more dramatic than to see somebody standing there with a body that is shaking all over and hands that are violently vibrating suddenly stop because the power of God has healed him. But that's exactly what happened.

A young man brought his mother to one of our services because she was suffering from severe headaches. The pain in her head was so severe that they shaved her head two and three times a week.

Whether it was the growing or the weight of the hair we do not know, but Frances laid hands on her and not knowing what else to do, she said, "In the name of Jesus, I command all of the electrical and chemical frequencies in every cell in your body to be in harmony and in balance and to digest the bad cells." Frances laid hands on her, and while she was going down under the power, she screamed, "I'm healed! No more pain!" It was an awesome and instant miracle. When she got up off of the floor, she could not believe what had happened to her in the twinkling of an eye. And that's all it takes with the power of God.

One of the most dramatic healings that we have ever seen occurred during a Saturday morning teaching session. I was ministering healing, and Frances was sitting on the stage when the pastor came up and whispered, "There's a girl here today who was accidently hit on the head with a large block of wood three years ago. It destroyed her equilibrium, and she has difficulty standing, walking, or doing anything." He said she had been in constant pain for three years and had been to every doctor, every chiropractor, and every clinic in the area, but they all told her exactly the same thing—that there was absolutely nothing that could be done for her.

She suffered pain twenty-four hours a day and was actually unable to do anything. She was one of the dancers in the ballet group in the church, but she had been unable to dance for three years.

There are times when you need to do more than one thing, so in her case the Holy Spirit spoke and told us to do two things. The first thing we did was to command the electrical and chemical frequencies in every cell in her body to be in harmony and in balance and to digest the bad cells. Then we did the "Nucca" on her. She was instantly, totally healed by the power of God. She stood there and, in the most beautiful, simple way, looked up and said, "I'm healed. I don't have any more pain."

Frances said, "If you are healed, then you will be able to dance." The musicians came up, and this woman who had been unable to do anything, even walking straight, for three years did the most beautiful ballet dance anyone could have ever seen. This was in her home church, and the church knew what her condition had been. The electricity of the Holy Spirit burst so upon the entire audience that they gave her an instant standing ovation, and every person in the house burst into tears. Thank You, Jesus, for that wonderful healing power.

Don't forget to command the electrical and chemical frequencies in every cell in your body to be in harmony and in balance and to digest the sick cells, in Jesus' name.

Do this command with any incurable disease, including blindness and deafness!

We use this command along with other suggested commands in all incurable diseases, and in any command where we feel it is needed.

It's very, very important!

Chapter Eight

Carpal Tunnel Syndrome

by Charles

Ministering healing is a constantly changing and improving opportunity. The more we minister healing, the more new ways we learn. We listen to medical doctors and chiropractors and have discovered innumerable successful ways to help people because new diseases and new "cures" crop up all the time. We often wonder if it is because people are living longer—which they are—or if it is because we have gone into more complicated jobs. Carpal tunnel syndrome is not one that is relegated to old age because it normally affects younger people, especially people who are computer operators, butchers, carpenters, hairdressers, or who work at any kind of a job that requires a tremendous amount of action in the wrist area.

Many times operators in these various jobs hold their hands or their fingers in the wrong position. Many computer operators hold their wrists down and their hands up and this often causes inflammation and swelling in that part of the wrist. Many of the flight attendants on airplanes who push carts, or those who do heavy work and heavy lifting with their wrists, discover that they have what the medical world calls carpal tunnel syndrome.

Recently a chiropractor told us about this common problem today among people who use their wrists a lot. It can cause such pain in the hand and wrist area that some individuals are unable to sleep or perform their work.

In the hinge of the wrist there exists a "tunnel" that houses ligaments and tendons. When the tunnel becomes inflamed or swollen through excessive use or misuse of the wrist, the passage is closed to varying degrees. Pain, weakness, or other discomforts in the wrist area arise. The ligaments or tendons may be stretched or jammed.

To heal carpal tunnel syndrome, place your thumb on one side of the soft spot in the wrist joint and a finger on the opposite side. Command the tunnel to open, both the inflammation and the swelling to be healed, and the tendons and ligaments to go back to normal length, position, and strength. Command them to be healed in the name of Jesus.

There is an extremely simple way to test for carpal tunnel syndrome. Have the person put his or her thumb and little finger together to form an O. Then put your forefinger in the circle and pull through the O. If the person has carpal tunnel syndrome, you can pull your finger through easily. Once it is healed, you won't be able to pull through the thumb and little finger.

Miracles for carpal tunnel syndrome happen regularly. Recently Frances had her hair done at a beauty parlor in preparation for having our pictures taken. Her hair stylist worked feverishly yet carefully to accomplish a perfect hairdo.

I noticed she wore a steel brace on her left wrist, extending about eight inches up her arm. When I asked her if she had carpal tunnel syndrome, she answered, "Yes." She added that she had taken care of sixty-two wigs that day.

Because of the strain this had put on her left hand, she could hardly move her wrist.

I asked her if she would like for God to heal it. The minute she got a break, I did what we had learned and gave the commands. We had tested the woman's strength, and there was no resistance when

I moved my finger through the loop she had made by holding her thumb and little finger in position. After we gave the commands, we immediately tested her strength again.

She was utterly amazed! She shook her wrist and in a few minutes had removed the brace. She was working free of pain. When we talked to her about two weeks later, she was exuberant with praise to God for completing this much-needed miracle.

A medical doctor recently called Frances to tell her his excitement about divine healing success after he watched our fifteen-hour video series and read the book *How to Heal the Sick*. She told him about carpal tunnel syndrome healings, explained to him how to test this before and after ministering, and how to do it.

About two weeks later this same physician called her again, but with even more excitement. He said many patients with carpal tunnel syndrome had come to him. Every single one was healed when he did what God had shown us. Then he asked with a laugh, "What should I do with the thousands of flyers I bought, telling how surgery could help heal the problem?"

WHAT ABOUT FEET?

A corresponding soft spot is located in the ankle area. Just in the bend of your ankle, beneath your ankle bone, you can have the same condition. This is called tarsal tunnel syndrome. This is healed exactly the same way as the wrist, although not nearly as many people have this problem as have carpal tunnel syndrome.

THE TARSAL TUNNEL

The tarsal tunnel contains the posterior tibial nerve and several blood vessels and tendons. It begins behind and above the ankle, moving around the inside of the ankle and into the bottom of the foot. If the nerve is damaged or compressed by trauma, swelling or growths surrounding tendons, blood vessels or bones, a painful condition called tarsal tunnel syndrome can result.

Each foot has twenty-six bones. This means that you have a great opportunity for a lot of those to get out of adjustment or out of place or turned because you're wearing the wrong shoes, or maybe because you have a weak ankle. You command the tunnel to open up and all the ligaments to be made whole in the name of Jesus.

On this one you could add, "In the name of Jesus, I command every bone in both feet to go into place and stay there."

TENDONITIS

Another ailment, tendonitis or "tennis elbow," is healed by the "carpal tunnel thing." If you will be alert to the nudgings of the Holy Spirit, you will discover many new ways to see someone healed.

Putting your thumb on one side of the wrist and your forefinger on the other, say, "In Jesus' name I command the carpal tunnel (or tarsal tunnel) to open and all ligaments and tendons to return to normal length and strength, and I command all pain and scar tissue to be healed."

Chapter Nine

Migraine Headaches and Tic Douloureux
(Trigeminal Neuralgia)

by Charles and Frances

Recently we visited with Hilton Sutton, president of Mission to America and a great Bible prophecy teacher. He shared with us for the first time that he had a problem called *tic douloureux,* or *trigeminal neuralgia.* We had seen only a few people healed of this painful affliction and did not know of any medical procedure that would help the problem.

The *American Medical Association Family Medical Guide,* published by Random House (New York,

1991), describes this affliction as pain from a damaged nerve.

This kind of neuralgia rarely affects anyone under fifty except in cases of multiple sclerosis. The trigeminal nerve is a major nerve in the face. If it is damaged, the result is severe pain that is usually felt on only one side of the face. Although it is not life-threatening, trigeminal neuralgia can be distressing and disabling.

We have talked to people who say it is one of the most painful afflictions there is. In fact, it is sometimes called the suicide disease. This same medical guide reports that the pain of trigeminal neuralgia shoots through one side of the face along the length of the nerve. It may last for a few seconds or as long as a minute or more. While it lasts it can be excruciating.

Sometimes attacks occur every few minutes for several days or weeks for no apparent reason. They may then fade, but stabbing pains usually return with decreasing intervals between them. Attacks may eventually become almost continuous. In some cases, occasional muscular spasms accompany the pain and cause a facial tic (twitching) or paralysis.

Hilton told us that for eight long and painful years he had suffered with tic douloureux. It was getting so bad that he was considering canceling some of his speaking engagements. Then he said, "The medical world has discovered a surgery that can stop this excruciating pain." We listened intently, because when a cause and a cure are discovered, we often find clues to a healing that God has in store for us.

He explained the type of surgery performed. They drill a hole through the skull into a place where a blood vessel or artery is too close to a nerve. Then they place a medical wedge between the two, which stops the pain.

Our response was "Thank You, Jesus!" Immediately we laid hands on Hilton's head and commanded divine wedges to separate the vessels or arteries and the nerve. We gave thanks to Jesus. When Hilton called a month later, he said the only pain he had experienced since that day was a headache resulting from a stressful situation.

Another month went by, and we talked again on the day we were writing this story. Hilton said he has had no more pain. Glory to God for healing him!

And thank You, Jesus, for showing us how to heal tic douloureux.

However, Hilton Sutton was so far behind on his work and his speaking engagements because of the excruciating pain of tic douloureux, when God healed him, he immediately started rebooking and overbooked himself including a long trip to Singapore and Malaysia. When he came back he was in the same condition he was in before God healed him. Hilton went to the hospital and had the operation done. The doctors worked for about four hours and said they'd never seen so many tangled nerves and blood vessels in their entire lives.

Hilton called us and said, "I know I was healed by God, but I brought it back on myself through over-work and through stress."

Stress is one of the worst things in the world to which any of us can subject ourselves because it brings on innumerable diseases. Hilton still maintains to this day that God healed him but he lost it through carelessness on his part.

The Bible says, "Cast all your cares on Him, and He will give you rest!" (See Matthew 11:28; 1 Peter 5:7.)

MIGRAINE HEADACHES

A man came to a three-day meeting. On the first day he said he had suffered most of his life with severe continual migraine headaches.

Led by God's Holy Spirit, we decided to do the same thing we had learned about tic douloureux. It worked! His headache immediately left and did not return the three days we were with him. In a follow-up call to him, he said how wonderful it was to live free of pain.

We have made the same command not only for migraine headaches, but also for other headaches.

Use this command: "In Jesus' name we command divine wedges to be driven between every vessel and nerve. Pain we rebuke you!"

Chapter Ten

The "Nucca"

by Charles and Frances

We learn new things all the time that really excite us. We believe if medical doctors and chiropractors can do it, we can do it with the power of God.

Following is an article that appeared in a magazine recently that has really taught us a lot about doing what we call "The Nucca Thing."

Is Your Head on Straight?
By Glenn Cripe, D.C.

Just when you thought you have tried everything, have you checked to see if your head is on straight?

Most people have experienced back pain or spinal-related problems sometime in their life. There are numerous approaches to achieving relief from this oftentimes disabling pain. There are procedures that vary as widely as bed rest to medications, acupuncture, acupressure, and then the extreme: surgery. All of these and other systems have had their degrees of successes and failures. Perhaps the one thing that can be said for certain is that there is no cure-all, no 100-percent solution for all back problems. It is, after all, a very complicated problem. The spinal column, various layers of muscles, and the nervous system largely make up the structure that not only allows us to remain upright under gravity, but also allows us to bend, twist, and tilt.

In seeking out help, most people will use the more conservative approaches first, like bed rest, and then keep moving toward the more extreme, like surgery, if they have not obtained the relief they need.

In this arena of back pain procedures, there is a system that offers still another approach. It's conservative, cost efficient, but, more importantly, extremely precise and painless. This procedure is named NUCCA after the National

Upper Cervical Chiropractic Association. The NUCCA principles were developed in Michigan by Drs. Ralph Gregory and John Grostic in the 1940s. NUCCA was formed in 1965 as a national organization recognized by the federal government. NUCCA is a specialty within the chiropractic profession that concentrates specifically on returning the head and neck to normal.

Most conditions that can benefit from chiropractic care usually begin and can end in the neck. Falls, a whiplash type of accident, or a twist of the neck can all result in the relationship of the head and neck going off center. By adjusting the head and neck, the entire spine, including the pelvis, can return back toward normal. This must be done before spinal balance can be attained.

The pelvis is the foundation for the spine; hence it supports the spine. As the head shifts off center, the pelvis must also shift. This is to keep the body as upright as possible. If the head is in its normal position, the pelvis will be directly under it. But if the head and neck misalign, the muscles of the back will automatically tighten to shift the pelvis so it will be as directly under the head as possible. This shifting of the structure of spine and pelvis can be the cause of many back problems, such as low back spasms, headaches, poor posture, or tingling pain in the extremities, etc. Unless the head and neck are returned back to their normal position, you may never really have a long-term correction with long-term results.

Because the pelvis is the supporting structure of the spine, NUCCA, through precise instrumentation, measures its displacement and uses it as a gauge in determining if the patient is in adjustment. Three very exacting X rays are taken and analyzed before any type of treatment is rendered. Each person has his or her unique type of misalignment pattern that must be precisely determined. Once the type and degree of misalignment have been established, the doctor is able to direct a slight and controlled pressure into the neck at a particular spot, which will then bring the head and neck back toward normal. The closer the doctor can restore the head and neck to normal, the more stable and long lasting the adjustment will be. As the body returns to normal, the muscles will pull evenly, relieving muscle spasms. Swelling around the nerves can subside, relieving the pinched nerve feeling. Postural changes can occur along with the removal of stress on the weight-bearing joints (hips, low back).

After the correction has taken place, both the doctor and patient should see significant results in postural changes. Within a three- to six-week period, symptomatic relief should occur.

Each case is unique, but generally symptoms can begin to alter from as soon as a few hours up to four to six weeks from the adjustment. After all, it usually has taken time to get out of shape. It will also take time for the tissue and nerves to heal.

As an alternative to correcting back problems, NUCCA has had wonderful results and research documented over the past forty-five years. So when you get to the point where you thought you've tried everything, you may want to find out if your head is on straight.

Dr. Glenn Cripe of Newport Beach is a Doctor of Chiropractics specializing in NUCCA.

The daughter of a friend of ours had twin babies a couple of years ago, and from the time of the delivery she had never been able to do any of her housework or the normal tasks associated with being a wife and a mother. She had been to many medical doctors and chiropractors and had received no relief whatsoever, until she found out about this NUCCA treatment. She went and had three treatments. After the third treatment, she was able to do normal housework, and she has remained healed ever since then.

We believe whatever can be done by a medical doctor or chiropractor can be done by using the power of God!

The first time we ever tried this was when a young man who had been in an automobile accident and was in excruciating pain in his back came to one of our services. We sat him down and measured his legs as we do when we do "The Leg Thing." He had one leg over four inches shorter than the other from this accident to his back. We did not do the usual "Leg Thing," but instead we laid our finger along his jawbone and made the command for the NUCCA. We said, "In the name of Jesus, we command the brain stem to be centered over the spine to relieve all problems in the back, and we command the brain stem and the head to line up perfectly with the spinal column."

After we had made this simple command in Jesus' name, we sat him down. His leg had grown out to absolute normal length with the other one, and he had no pain whatsoever! He spent the rest of the night rejoicing and praising God. What a thrill to see this work the first time we tried it.

We have done this many times since then with remarkable success.

If you will look at the diagrams on pages 92–93, you will see what happens before and after an accident, and it doesn't have to be an automobile accident. It can be any kind where the body is stretched abnormally.

Put your finger on the top vertebra (first bone of the spine). Then speak this command: "In Jesus' name I command the head and neck to move into the position so that every vertebra and disc go into perfect alignment and be healed from top to bottom!"

If this does not completely alleviate the pain, then do "TTT."

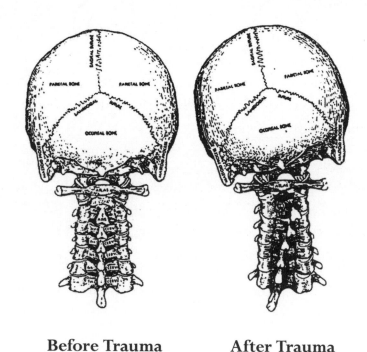

Before Trauma   **After Trauma**

Here's what happens before trauma and after trauma: Prior to a spinal trauma, the twelve-pound head is evenly centered over the neck. After the trauma, the head has shifted away from center. To compensate, the neck buckles from its intended position, putting undue stress on muscles and ligaments.

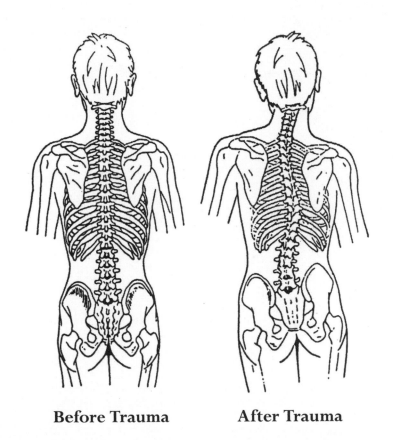

Before Trauma   **After Trauma**

The spinal column remains straight and balanced as long as the head is centered over the neck. Following an accident, the head is shifted away from center. To compensate for the change and to keep the body in balance, the entire spinal column begins to buckle. Over time, an injury to the head and neck can cause low back pain.

Chapter Eleven

When Ministering Healing

by Charles and Frances

This *Handbook for Healing,* along with the book and video and audio tapes called *How to Heal the Sick,* can only briefly and simply teach basic principles of healing. In no sense is this to be considered all-inclusive or to indicate any application of medical or scientific procedures or practices. These are only suggested guidelines.

We urge everyone who possibly can to study our video tapes and books, plus the doctors' panels videos. Much can be learned from them. The principles of applying the healing methods outlined in the

Bible and in our teachings will be imprinted on your mind. Audio tapes of the various Healing Explosion doctors' panels are available through our office and are very valuable teachings.

If you desire further information about various diseases, many good medical dictionaries and handbooks are available through bookstores. If in doubt, ask your doctor to help you. Also do a search on the Internet.

We can never repeat often enough that you follow the advice of your doctor. We are not doctors, and we urge all believers to never try to follow medical procedures, but simply to do the childlike application of God's power in Jesus' name.

AIDS: Acquired Immune Deficiency Syndrome

We want to include a word about AIDS, or Acquired Immune Deficiency Syndrome. This particular disease is presented in detail since it is such a devastating problem, and because the incidence is rapidly on the rise in our day and time. In April 1987, we were told that there was no medical cure for AIDS, no prospective cure, and little hope for an effective vaccine. Since then, there is still no cure—only medications that help people with the disease to live longer. The Christian community has seen more and more people requesting ministering of healing for this disease.

What is AIDS? This is a disease caused by a virus called HTLV-III, or the AIDS virus.

What does it do? The AIDS virus causes a severe reduction and depletion of the immune system of a person until his or her body can no longer effectively fight off infection.

How is the virus transmitted? The primary way in which the AIDS virus is passed from one person to another is through sexual intercourse. It was first thought that only homosexual contact was transmitting the disease, but now it is clear that people with multiple heterosexual contacts are also at risk. This obviously means that the person married to someone with AIDS is at risk of developing the disease as well.

AIDS can also be passed through blood transfusions, and through the use of dirty hypodermic needles. It could possibly also be passed from an open sore or bleeding cut into an open cut or mucous membrane of another person. There is suspicion, but no evidence, that intense kissing may transfer the virus. There is also no evidence that any casual contact, like shaking hands, a kiss on the cheek, or sneezing or coughing can infect others.

How do I minister to someone with AIDS? If the person contracted the disease through either homosexual or promiscuous activity, the first thing he needs to do is repent and be born again. We firmly believe there will never be a healing of AIDS without complete and genuine repentance and a turning away from the lifestyle in which one has previously been engaged.

The plan of salvation is extremely important in the healing of this particular disease, so don't rush over this part of the healing.

Then rebuke and take authority over the infection in the name of Jesus, and cast out the spirit of AIDS in Jesus' name. Command healing or restoration to the entire immune system in the name of Jesus. Command the entire body to be healed and restored to normal in the name of Jesus. Also do the "electrical and chemical frequencies thing."

The root cause of AIDS still stems from sins that are abominations to God. An innocent spouse or individual may get AIDS and not be guilty of sin himself, but the source still seems to descend from the sin.

Here are a few Scriptures that clearly tell what God thinks about this sin against the body, which is intended to be His temple:

All of Leviticus 18 deals with the laws of sexual morality. Specifically, verses 22, 24, and 29 in the *New King James Version* say,

> *You shall not lie with a male as with a woman. It is an abomination....Do not defile yourselves with any of these things....For whoever commits any of these abominations, the persons who commit them shall be cut off from among their people.*

We also find the following passages in Leviticus and 1 Corinthians, respectively:

> *If a man lies with a male as he lies with a woman, both of them have committed an abomination. They shall surely be put to death. Their blood shall be upon them.*
> (Leviticus 20:13 NKJV)

> *Do you not know that the unrighteous will not inherit the kingdom of God? Do not be deceived. Neither fornicators, nor idolaters, nor adulterers, nor homosexuals, nor sodomites, nor thieves, nor covetous, nor drunkards, nor revilers, nor extortioners will inherit the kingdom of God. And such were some of you. But you were washed, but you were sanctified, but you were justified in the name of the Lord Jesus and by the Spirit of our God.* (1 Corinthians 6:9–11 NKJV).

Praise God for the redemption plan of Jesus! Is there hope for healing people with AIDS? Yes—in Jesus!

DRINK PLENTY OF WATER

We listened to a Trinity Broadcasting Network (TBN) program recently where there were eight doctors and two nutritionists, and they all said that the problem with the sick body of Christ is that none of us are drinking enough water.

We constantly get information about what water does, but recently we received an e-mail that contained some interesting facts. We're going to pass the information on to you and hope that you will start drinking more water.

Seventy-five percent of Americans are chronically dehydrated (likely applies to half the world population).

In 37 percent of Americans, the thirst mechanism is so weak that it is often mistaken for hunger.

Even *mild* dehydration will slow down one's metabolism as much as 3 percent.

One glass of water shut down midnight hunger pangs for almost 100 percent of the dieters studied in a University of Washington study.

Lack of water is the number one trigger of daytime fatigue.

Preliminary research indicates that eight to ten glasses of water a day could significantly ease back and joint pain for up to 80 percent of sufferers.

A mere 2 percent drop in body water can trigger fuzzy short-term memory, trouble with basic math, and difficulty focusing on the computer screen or on a printed page.

Drinking five glasses of water daily decreases the risk of colon cancer by 45 percent, plus it can slash the risk of breast cancer by 79 percent, and one is 50 percent less likely to develop bladder cancer.

Are you drinking the amount of water you should every day?

MINISTERING TO CHILDREN

When ministering to children, remember that you are much bigger than they are, and if you are not careful, you may frighten them and lose their confidence.

This principle also applies to adults, especially to those who have never been exposed to divine healing or deliverance. Be careful to approach them in gentleness and love. You may be "full grown" in the supernatural, while they may be as little children, and there is also a risk of frightening them and losing their confidence.

One of the best ways to approach a child is to come down to their level by kneeling. It helps a great deal to always smile and talk to them quietly and confidently. One good way to gain contact with a youngster is to extend your hands to them, palms upward and open, so they can place their hands in yours.

While ministering to them, do not raise your voice. It is possible to continue smiling at the youngster at the same time you are taking authority over an evil spirit and casting it out in Jesus' name. Speak with authority, and that spirit will recognize that you mean business, and it will obey. A child will always recognize when someone is ministering in love, and he will respond. Therefore, project to him from the inside of you that you love him and you are there to help him.

MENTAL ILLNESS

How an individual thinks is a result of what he or she has allowed into the mind. Therefore, when the wrong thoughts and thought patterns come across the mind, regardless of their origin, it is up to each individual to either receive, reject, or replace them with the right thinking and thought pattern.

It has been said that practically all mental illness is the result of guilt. If so, that simply means there is sin in the life. To gain control and mastery of that area requires an acknowledgment by that person of the problem source, a genuine repentance, with a turning away from sin, and an acceptance of Jesus Christ as Lord and Savior.

Insanity is classified as mental illness as we discuss it here.

To minister healing, first bind and cast out the spirit of whatever the problem is: depression, oppression, schizophrenia, mania, and so on, by the power of the Holy Spirit, in Jesus' name. Next speak the peace of God into that mind and heart in the name of Jesus.

Since a major part of the problem originated in wrong thinking, then the most important step is to change the thinking by renewing the mind (see Romans 12:1–2) by filling the mind and the life with the Word of God. The Word says, *"Let this mind be in you which was also in Christ Jesus"* (Philippians 2:5 NKJV).

Notice that it is a choice that we must make; God will not do it for us. We are to renew our minds with God's Word by reading it, meditating on it, confessing it, occupying our minds with it, and living it, until we begin to think the same way God thinks.

People need to be delivered, saved, and baptized in the Holy Spirit, and then they need to get into the Word of God.

Then, the only way for them to remain free of this bondage is to obey Jesus and be doers of the Word. That means they must put the desires and purposes of God and Jesus above their own. Those who look inward will perish in darkness, but those whose light shines outward to reveal Jesus will remain free.

> *Therefore if the Son makes you free, you shall be free indeed.*   (John 8:36 NKJV)

SUICIDE

People who have a tendency toward suicide really need help, and it is best to realize that while some of them need deliverance from demonic powers, others are caught in deep feelings of defeat and depression. Tell them that God loves them and He has provided a way for them to be free, if they will just ask Jesus to forgive them and to come into their heart.

In a firm but quiet voice, with power and authority, look into their eyes and cast out the spirit: "Devil, I bind you in the name of Jesus and by the power of the Holy Spirit, and I command you, spirit of suicide, to come out of this person now in Jesus' name."

Minister salvation and the baptism with the Holy Spirit to give them power to live victoriously.

Urge them to get into a good church under the ministry of Spirit-filled pastors. They need to learn how to look outward and help others, for only as we give can we receive.

Chapter Twelve

The Spine

D r. Roy J. LeRoy has been at all of our Healing Explosions. He is an outstanding chiropractor who actively practiced in his field for forty years before he retired. He shared his valuable knowledge and experience with us on the doctors' panels at Healing Explosions. We suggest that you view our video tapes of the panels.

Norma Jean Van Dell, about whom we wrote the book, *Impossible Miracles,* was widowed, but God sent a widower to sweep her off her feet, and she became Mrs. LeRoy in 1984. Their joint ministry to the sick is entitled Impossible Miracles Ministry and is a powerful, unique ministry.

Recently something Doc said triggered a great response in us. We feel it will be a real blessing to you.

> All bitterness and resentment start first with anger. Somebody does something to you that makes you angry. This causes an overabundance of adrenalin to be supplied into your body. The body cannot absorb the excess amount of adrenalin that shoots out, and as a result it goes into the kidneys, but they are unable to carry off this excess. It has to go someplace, so it settles in the joints of the body, which causes arthritis.

We would wholeheartedly recommend to anybody who has arthritis that you look deeply in your life and see if you have bitterness and unforgiveness toward another person. If so, get it out of your system.

This is not the only cause of arthritis according to statistics, but is one of the most significant.

Dr. LeRoy has blessed our healing teams mightily in his knowledge of the spine, and he has provided the following for your benefit.

THE SPINE

by Dr. Roy J. LeRoy

It is estimated that close to 85 percent of adults will have back and/or neck problems of some sort during their lifetime. Most of these problems are a result of some kind of injury. Usually the condition that occurs is a combination of misaligned vertebrae, muscle strain, ligament and tendon strain or tearing. In addition, the disc that sits between the vertebrae may also be damaged.

With this high incidence of spinal problems, a large percentage of people who come for healing will have this as their complaint. Charles and Frances have given nicknames to these ways of ministering healing. Almost all of these problems are ministered to by:

- "Growing out arms" (the arm thing)

- "Growing out legs" (the leg thing)

- The neck thing (TNT), and/or

- The pelvic thing (TPT)

They call the combination of all of these "The total thing" (TTT).

Therefore, we will briefly review the spine and its problems.

The vertebrae are the bones that make up the spinal column, sitting one on top of the other. In between these vertebrae are the discs, or pads, that allow a certain amount of motion in bending and twisting the back and neck. All of these bones are held in place by sets of ligaments, tendons, and muscles. In the back the vertebral column is a channel made up of the circular rings of bone on the back of the vertebrae that house and protect the spinal cord, the main bundle of nerves running from the brain to all the parts of the body.

A severe fracture or dislocation can cause damage to the cord itself, or to any of the thirty-one pairs of nerve roots that come out from between the individual vertebrae. Damage to a disc, the pad between the vertebrae, can cause it to bulge out and put pressure on a nerve root, causing pain and at times weakness on either one side or both sides of the body.

The spine starts just under the base of the skull with what is called the cervical spine. This is the series of the first seven vertebrae, the topmost being the Atlas and the second one the Axis. The head rotates from side to side on the Atlas, and forward and backward on the Axis.

The nerves from the cervical spine supply the face and head, the neck, shoulders, and partway down the arms. Any pressure on these nerves will cause pain and interference with normal function in these areas. For healing in this area we do "the neck thing."

The thoracic (or dorsal) spine consists of the next twelve vertebrae, each of which has a pair of ribs coming off the sides, forming the rib cage. The nerves that come out from the spinal cord at this level supply the lower arms, the hands, and the chest. For healing in this area, we do what is called "growing out arms."

The lumbar spine consists of the bottom five vertebrae, where the nerves supplying the legs and feet come from between the vertebrae. For healing in this area we do what is called "growing out legs."

The next bone, rather larger than the vertebrae, is called the sacrum, and supplies support for the entire spinal column. This bone is also joined to the two hip, or iliac, bones (a part of the pelvis) through a series of ligaments, tendons, and the sacroiliac joints. For ministering healing to the entire pelvic area, we do what is called "the pelvic thing." The thigh bones, or femurs, are joined to the hip bones.

Just below the sacrum is the coccyx bone, a short bone that comes close to the rectum, also known as the tailbone.

While ministering to someone with a neck or back injury, it is not uncommon to find that they have been to a doctor and may be wearing an orthopedic collar or brace. Do not remove or readjust the apparatus when ministering, since this could be considered practicing medicine. After the person has been ministered to, we suggest that you ask him if the pain is gone. Normally he can tell whether there has been improvement while the collar or brace is still in place. If he report thats the problem has improved, you may ask him if *he* wants to remove the apparatus to see what God has done. Let it be his choice.

Encourage the person to return to his doctor for evaluation, qualification, or verification as appropriate.

PINCHED NERVES

In the diagram on the following page are listed a few of the many problems, disorders, and diseases that pinched nerves can cause in the various areas of the body.

The arrows on the left point to the locations in the spine where nerves pass through very small openings on their way to and from the brain to control all the various parts and organs of the body. About 300,000 nerve fibers pass through each of the sixty-two little openings. Just a slight dislocation of a bone (vertebra) in the spine can close one of these tiny openings enough to pinch a nerve and interfere with normal passage of nerve impulses.

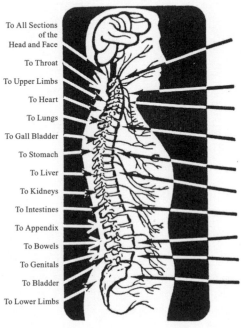

To All Sections of the Head and Face

To Throat

To Upper Limbs

To Heart

To Lungs

To Gall Bladder

To Stomach

To Liver

To Kidneys

To Intestines

To Appendix

To Bowels

To Genitals

To Bladder

To Lower Limbs

1. Dizziness, headaches, nervousness, eye and ear problems, high blood pressure, chronic tiredness, migraine headaches, nervous breakdown, insomnia, fainting spells, glandular troubles, allergies.

2. Skin disorders, hay fever, wry or stiff neck, neuralgia, neuritis, sore throat, hoarseness.

3. Bronchial conditions, throat conditions, arm and shoulder pain, bursitis, asthma, coughs, thyroid conditions.

4. Pain and numbness in forearms and hands, chest pains, congestion, palpitation, "nervous" or fast heart, pleurisy.

5. Gall bladder problems, jaundice, shingles, stomach upsets, heartburn, fever.

6. Low blood pressure, poor circulation, ulcers, hives, stomach trouble.

7. Hiccoughs, lowered resistance, dyspepsia, circulatory problems, rheumatism.

8. Certain types of sterility, impotence, menstrual troubles, diarrhea, constipation.

9. Knee pains, varicose veins, prostate problems, bed wetting, backaches, cold feet.

10. Poor circulation, leg cramps, hemorrhoids, ankle swelling, rectal itching, pain on sitting.

Chapter Thirteen

The "Appestat"

by Mary Ruth Swope

D r. Mary Ruth Swope received her B.S. degree from Winthrop College in Rockville, South Carolina. She then went on to receive her Master of Science degree, including nutrition, from the University of North Carolina at Greensboro.

Her doctorate is from the Columbia University in New York City. She taught high school for seven years, then worked as a nutritionist for the Ohio Health Department for three years. Dr. Swope then entered the college arena, where she was a member of the Foods and Nutrition Faculty at Purdue University, and later served as Head of Foods and Nutrition at the University of Nevada.

For eighteen years prior to her retirement in December 1980, Dr. Swope was Dean of the School of Home Economics, Eastern Illinois University, Charleston, Illinois.

Well qualified in the field of nutrition, Dr. Mary Ruth Swope has made excellent contributions to the Healing Explosions (as you can see on our videos). She attended almost every Healing Explosion, and her advice is excellent and up-to-date.

She is a specialist in the area of the "appestat," as she calls it, and shares some of her wealth of knowledge in this area on the following pages.

DEFINITION OF APPESTAT

The appestat is the appetite control center in the hypothalmus gland in the brain. It is regulated by the blood sugar level. Compare it to the thermostat in your house. When the air cools off, the furnace comes on until the temperature cuts off the thermostat. That's the way the appestat works, except that our junk-food and high-sugar diet has "broken" the appestat. God needs to repair it by readjusting the set-point. God uses you to do that by the laying on of hands and by your command.

SPIRITUAL ASPECTS OF THE OBESITY PROBLEM

Overweight people are often harassed by the following:

1. Addiction to sugar, fats, salt, junk foods, etc.
2. Gluttony
3. Caffeine
4. Craving for unwholesome drinks (ale, beer, bourbon, brandy, champagne, soft drinks, wine, etc.)
5. Craving for unwholesome foods (pork, shrimp, catfish, etc.)
6. Morbid hunger—hunger experiences shortly after a meal, which results in bulimia
7. Inheritance bonds
8. Deception of overeating (lust for food)
9. Anxiety or insecurity
10. Fear of not getting enough to eat in the presence of plenty

God has promised to guide you, even in the details of situations. He knows what you need to do and say. You may not! Trust Him to act on your behalf and that of the people who are to receive deliverance and healing.

When praying for people, put one hand on their forehead. God will become their nutrition teacher and will show them what to eat and not to eat. Lay your other hand on their appestat at the base of their brain. God will reset their "out-of-control" appestats. They will glorify God through controlled body weight, if they obey Him.

Miracle after miracle will take place before your eyes. God's Spirit will be working in marvelous and miraculous ways.

Pray much for obese people. I will show you that is what they need. Healing of the appetite is no different than healing a kneecap or some other dysfunctioning part of the body. Illness to any part, no matter how small or inconsequential it seems, can destroy the whole being. Appetite is no exception.

Divine healing of the appestat will bring normalcy to the dietary pattern, and when eating habits return to normal, bodies heal themselves to a great extent.

Overnutrition of the body is often accompanied by undernutrition of the spirit and soul. People get fat, bloated, and often forget their God as the Israelites did! Science cannot solve this problem. That's obvious. But God can! Jesus will set the captives free through the laying on of hands.

Almost nobody in Christendom has had the vision of the devil's sneaky plan to destroy health, wealth, and happiness through diet manipulation. That is why Christians are overeating, overfed, and overweight. *Millions* are headed for beds of affliction accompanied by high medical bills. They have not stopped to think how this affects God's marching army, His supply of soldiers, in these last days.

See obesity as a destroyer, a killer. Gluttony maims! Millions will attest to this fact. Abnormal excesses result in specific diseases that destroy the body, the soul, and the spirit. See yourself as a partial answer to this problem.

Speak to the person to whom you are ministering, without condemnation, and ask him to pray with you.

SUGGESTED PRAYER

In the name of Jesus, I speak to my body and command my thoughts about food to line up with good nutrition. I bind any spirit of lust for sugar, fat, pork, blood, too much meat, junk foods, and all other unhealthful foods.

I speak to my body and command my metabolism to become perfectly normal. Digestive organs, I command you to work as they were meant to work, in the name of Jesus.

I speak to my "appestat" and command it to be healed at the upper limits, in the name of Jesus. I will no longer experience a ferocious appetite or be tempted to go on eating binges.

I say, appetite, that you will learn to love pleasant bread, and you will eat it willingly, without murmuring—for the glory of God and the sake of the kingdom, in the name of Jesus. Amen.

"For God is at work within you, helping you want to obey him, and then helping you do what he wants" (Philippians 2:13 TLB).

SUGAR: THE INFLICTOR OF GREAT PUNISHMENT

A noted doctor said, "Sugar is the greatest scourge (a whip that inflicts great punishment) that has ever been visited on man in the name of food." He believes that it should be outlawed as a poison, because that's what it is. It has perverted our appetites and ruined our internal organs. It is supplying the perfect food for our cancer, heart trouble, diabetes, soft bones, pancreatitis, kidney disease, liver disease, sticky blood platelets, and dental caries; and it increases our desire for coffee and alcohol. He suggests that when you substitute dextrose and any other kind of sugar for white table sugar, it is comparable to exchanging a rattlesnake for a cobra as a bed partner!

Endocrinologists agree that sugar destroys God's relative balance of the glands and nervous system. These are the glands that produce and secrete hormones into the blood or lymph, to all parts of the body.

Sugar upsets the balance and produces a hypersecretion of hormones comparable to what you get with taking drugs and artificial hormones. In addition, it is addictive.

One of the most damaging things is that it causes the appetite control center to go helter-skelter. Sugar is devoid of any nutritional value (except calories), so the cells do not get the vitamins, minerals, enzymes, protein, and so on, that they need.

When you ingest sugar, the "sugar glands" go to work, telling you to eat more food so that your cells might have a chance to get the missing nutrients for which they are looking. Your pancreas works harder to provide more insulin. It tells your brain to eat more sugar because it cannot slow down fast enough to keep from throwing you into a coma. So, you receive double damage—you eat more junk, and your glands keep working to tell you to give them more nutrients!

A recent study, in which people ate eighteen hundred calories per day of sweet foods, reported up to a 40 percent increase in cholesterol in two weeks. The most frightening finding was that table sugar was found in the urine of all participants.

As one doctor said, "It remains to be seen what the twenty-first century people will be like; their endocrine glands are going to be damaged from birth. Heart disease will be up, even from birth; we are seeing children born now with plugged blood vessels, especially boy babies.

WHO WILL PROTECT US FROM THIS DESTRUCTION?

Will dieticians? No, they give you Jello, which has 60 percent sugar in it, right after you've been assaulted by a surgeons' knife!

Will home economics teachers? No, they are still teaching young people to bake the richest, sweetest cookies, cakes, puddings, and so on, that you can imagine.

Will food manufacturers? No, sugar is cheap, and sugar sells products. So they will find new ways to foist more sugar on us. Filled, iced, and fried doughnuts will attest to that!

A noted doctor says that we are headed for nutritional obliteration. The devil loves it! God hates it! It was never His plan for man to destroy himself through poor nutrition.

GOD'S ANSWER VERSUS SATAN'S COUNTERFEIT

God's Answer: Honey	Satan's Counterfeit: Sugar
"My son, eat honey because it is good, and the honeycomb which is sweet to your taste" (Proverbs 24:13 NKJV). *"It is not good to eat much honey; so to seek one's own glory is not glory"* (Proverbs 25:27 NKJV).	*"For what purpose to Me comes...sweet cane from a far country?"* (Jeremiah 6:20 NKJV).

1. Contains at least fifteen nutrients; an excellent food.	1. No nutrients. A *poison*. Not a food.
2. In a raw state, is an aid to digestion because of enzyme content.	2. Sugar in the stomach causes fermentation and putrefication and interference with digestion.
3. In moderation, does not adversely affect immune system.	3. Completely breaks down immune system, causing many disease conditions to flourish.
4. A natural antibiotic.	4. Causes fermentation, leading to bacterial growth and many diseases.
5. Satisifies appetite; does not interfere with desire for nourishing food.	5. Causes gluttony and craving for more sweets.
6. In moderation, does not contribute to weight gain.	6. One of the main causes of excess weight.
7. Enters bloodstream slowly and perfectly (two calories per minute).	7. Produces a yo-yo effect.
8. In moderation, is not harmful to the joints.	8. Contributes to arthritis.
9. Useful to alcoholics when recovering.	9. Excess sugar contributes to alcoholism.
10. Is psychologically and emotionally satisfying.	10. Causes mental disturbances, nervous disorders, and stress.

11. Does not destroy bone structure.

11. Causes calcium leakage from bones, resulting in osteoporosis.

12. Does not contribute to heart disease, heart attacks, strokes, or high blood pressure.

12. Causes heart disease and high blood pressure.

13. Does not cause distortion of vision.

13. Dims and blurs vision and can cause double vision (your eyes are what you eat).

THE BOTTOM LINE

Sugar contributes to a diseased state of health and often results in a shortened lifespan.

Chapter Fourteen

Eye Healings

by Dr. Burton J. Dupuy, Jr.

Dr. Burton J. Dupuy, Jr., an optometrist from Natchitoches, Louisiana, attended the New Orleans healing seminar, and the information he shared with us resulted in more eye healings than in all of our other Healing Explosions put together. The results continue, so we pass this information on to you.

There are two eye problems that you will probably run into most often. They are glaucoma and cataracts.

Some people say these eye problems are inherited. You might ask the person if anyone in his family has one of these diseases or situations. They are not necessarily inherited.

Cataracts are due to poor circulation, I believe, more than anything else. We're not really sure what causes it, but we do know that a lack of oxygen supply to the lens in the eye will cause cataracts. Some are spots, some are streaks, some are like dust on the cornea, some are just milky—there are all types. Pray that the spot in the eye will be removed. Command the spirit of inheritance to come out.

A cataract is not a growth. The lens in the eye where the cataract is formed is shaped like a magnifying lens. It is thick in the middle and thin on the edges. It is composed of layer after layer of skin, similar to an onion. What happens is these layers start drying out in different areas, and this causes a spot. So when the light comes through, when we look into the eye, we see a black spot in there. It is not a growth; it is not cancerous. It is just a change or drying out of the tissue. Pray that the tissue will be restored to normal and the blood supply to the eye will be replenished.

Glaucoma is an increase of pressure in the eye. The fluids in the eye are constantly being replaced and drained out. The canals are slim around the outer area of the iris where the fluids drain out of the eye, and if these canals become clogged, then the drainage slows down and the pressure builds up. It's like blowing air into a balloon. Command the canals to be opened, command the spirit of inheritance to come out, and command the pressure to be relieved and go down to normal, in Jesus' name.

Chapter Fifteen

The Difference between a Miracle and a Healing

by Frances

We all wish that we could lay hands on the sick and see them instantly recover. We love it when we lay hands on a person who has palsy, make a command in the name of Jesus, and then see them stop shaking immediately. This awesome miracle recently happened to us.

A lady got in the wrong line, and Charles laid hands on her for diabetes. When she fell under the power I said, "Charles, no, that's not diabetes; that's Parkinson's disease." So while she was on the floor, we made the electrical and chemical frequency command that we talked about in chapter seven. She looked right up at us and said, "I'm healed because I stopped shaking." She got up off of the floor and held her arms up in the air. Where she had been violently shaking before, there was not even a slight tremor!

This brought the whole audience to their feet in a standing ovation to Jesus because it was the first healing of the evening. It was a special time! How we all wish they could all be like this!

A lady came to a recent meeting of ours and said she had been in an automobile accident thirty-six years ago. For thirty-six years she had suffered excruciating pain day and night with no relief. She said she had slept very little in the thirty-six years because the pain was so intense. She had been to medical doctors, she had been to chiropractors, she had been to every source you could think of, and she said, "I have not lived in thirty-six years. I have just existed." Her face showed the pain that she had been through.

A simple command was made, and how we wish there had been a camera to catch the expression on her face! She was totally shocked to discover that suddenly (and that's how quickly it happened) the pain disappeared 100 percent. She bent over; she ran; she walked up and down stairs; she did everything you could think of, and there was not one sign of pain left in her body!

These are the kinds of healings we wish happened all the time. Don't get discouraged when they don't happen, but be excited when they do.

A little boy came to our service with rheumatoid arthritis. He was nine years old, and his parents told us he had never had a day without pain. This is really difficult on a child because it made it impossible for him to play or participate in any games with other children. But their great faith brought him hundreds of miles to come to the service. His healing was quick, because children are easily healed since their faith is so simple. We made the usual command for rheumatoid arthritis, and suddenly he looked up with simple childlike faith and said, "Do you know I don't have any pain in my body at all?"

He immediately began feeling his knees and feeling his feet and feeling his hands. He looked at me and said, "I don't have anything. I don't have a bit of pain anywhere!" Then he took off and ran down the aisle of the church to tell his mother that the pain was all gone.

This is the kind that, of course, excites the person prayed for, the person who did the praying, and an entire congregation! How we wish all healings would be that way, and we believe someday they will! The instant one is the miracle healing!

But there is another wonderful kind of healing that takes place over time. Many people, when they come forward, are praying and hoping and expecting their healing to be an instant healing. But what happens if they don't get healed immediately?

Don't let the devil steal your healing from you! The power of God has gone into the person prayed for, and the power of God will continue to work in him! Many people, if they do not get an instant healing, make the mistake of going back to their seat and saying immediately, "I didn't get my healing." This is allowing the devil to steal what happened to you, so don't ever listen when the devil tells you that. When we're laying hands on the sick, we need to encourage people to continue to believe for their healing.

There has been a lot of comments, both pro and con, by some people in the Word Faith movement, which taught that all you have to say is, "By His stripes I am healed," and you will be healed. This has worked for many people, and we don't want to discourage you from standing on the Word of God. Our pastor, John Osteen, taught his congregation an incredible truth that we think helps a lot in this situation.

Romans 4:17 says that we can call into being those things which do not exist as though they did, but Pastor John said, "You cannot call the things that are as though they are not." In other words, if you have cancer, you cannot stand up and say, "I do not have cancer in my body." The provision for your healing is there, but you are not healed until you are healed. You cannot deny that you have cancer.

At this point, we really want to share something right from our hearts. Once in a while you will pray for healing, but you don't get healed, and the condition worsens and worsens until something has to be done. Don't get upset.

Several years ago I had to have an artificial knee replacement in my right leg. I believed up to the very last minute that God was going to give me a new kneecap, and I even insisted before I went to surgery that the doctor take a last-minute X ray. But God did not put in a new one.

Now what should I have done? I had believed for my healing, but I didn't get it. I have more new parts than I have original parts, but the knee was not one of them. I didn't intend to hobble around crippled the rest of my life, so I just said, "Thank You, Jesus," and we asked God to guide the surgeon's hand. I did not say, "I have received a new knee." I suppose I could have said that, because up until that time I had been walking bone on bone, and it really hurt. But when I had the knee replacement put in, the pain totally disappeared. I did have a new knee, but not the kind I had expected.

Well, Frances, aren't you ashamed to tell people that you had to have a knee replacement? No! God can take any mess and make a miracle out of it. The doctor who did the surgery accepted Jesus as His Savior and Lord. When people heard I was in the hospital, they came into my room, and we were able to minister healing to them. We also were able to put our video tapes on *How to Heal the Sick* in the doctor's waiting room. Hallelujah!

So you see, if you have to submit to an operation, you'll get your healing one way or another. You might say, "Well, you didn't get healed because you lacked faith."

I don't know why God works the way He does; ask Him. I don't understand why I didn't get a new knee. I don't understand why I did get a new heart supernaturally.

Let me explain healing in this way. Most of us have a thermostat in our house. Sometimes we need our house to be cooler, and sometimes we need it to be a little warmer. When you come in from the cold and it's snowing outside, your thermostat might be set at sixty degrees, and it feels as cold as can be in your house. What is the first thing you do? You go to the thermostat and turn it up. Now, what is the second thing you do? If it doesn't immediately jump to seventy-two degrees, do you kick the thermostat and say, "Well, it doesn't work. I'll just break that thing because it doesn't work"?

No, that's not what you do at all. You are perfectly content to wait until the temperature goes up, and we all know that it takes a little time to get a thermostat from sixty up to seventy-two degrees. So all we do is patiently wait.

The same thing is true of healings. Sometimes you get an instant healing, but sometimes you have to wait. Sometimes healings can take place over a twenty-four-hour period. Sometimes it might even take a month or two before the healing is complete. But we always recommend to people that they keep thanking Jesus for the healing while it is going on. Don't let the devil come in and rob you with doubt and unbelief about your healing. Rather, keep thanking God and saying, "Thank You, Jesus; I know my healing is on the way."

If I were you, right now I would set my thermostat at seventy-two degrees for whatever is wrong with your body. If you're down to fifty or forty degrees, it might take you a little while to get up to seventy-two, but remember that you are on the way.

Dodie Osteen's book, *Healed of Cancer,* is a must for everyone who is battling cancer. Here is an excerpt:

Dodie was diagnosed on Thursday, December 10, 1981. John Osteen was told the following devastating news. The doctor said, "Pastor, your wife has metastatic cancer of the liver. With or without chemotherapy, she has only a few weeks to live. We can treat her, but it will only slightly prolong her life.

"However, we cannot find the primary tumor," he said. "We don't know where it is. In fact, it has really baffled us. Usually a primary tumor signifies the beginning of cancer and then it spreads to the liver or kidneys or some place else. But we cannot find one. With your consent, we would like to do exploratory surgery or a colonoscopy to try to locate the tumor."

John couldn't believe it. He said, "Doctor, I am going to take my wife home. We are going to pray and seek God, and then we will decide what to do. We believe in miracles, and we believe in the Miracle Worker."

The doctor said, "Well, Pastor, you're going to have to have a miracle this time."

Dodie went home on December 10, 1981, and never went back to the hospital. John anointed her with oil the day after she got home from the hospital. As they were both on the floor in their bedroom, face down before God, he took authority over any disease and over all cancerous cells in her body.

Dodie said, "As far as I'm concerned, that's the day my healing began." Dodie fought the symptoms and the attacks of the devil for five years—five long years, but her faith never wavered. Even though it was not an instant miracle, it started on the day when she and John made a covenant that her healing had begun. Today, many years later, she is a beautiful woman, a picture of health.

One of my favorite stories about Dodie Osteen's healing is this:

> When I was sick, I would look at two pictures of me in radiant health—one in my wedding dress and one riding a horse on a ranch. They bolstered my faith and helped me keep a positive attitude— especially when I was feeling so sick.
>
> I kept looking at those pictures and saying, "Thank You, Father, that You will restore health to me and heal me of my wounds. I thank You that I'll feel like I did when I married at twenty-one. I'll feel like I did when I was twenty-five,

riding that horse. I thank You that You will restore me to health, Father."

When I started feeling good again, I said, "Father, thank You that You have restored health to me." I repeat this often—even now!

It was a miracle of God regardless of how you look at it!

Don't get discouraged if you don't see an instant miracle. Some miracles happen the moment you lay hands on the sick, but other healings take time. Tell the person to whom you are ministering that the healing power went into him once you have laid hands on him. Do everything you can to keep people from becoming discouraged. Build their faith—and yours—with every sentence you speak.

We do not lay hands on the sick when we feel like it. We lay hands on the sick at every opportunity! Some of the greatest healings we have ever seen have taken place when we were sick or completely exhausted. Don't wait for a feeling—do it now!

When God opens a door for you, go through it. He always has something special for you on the other side. Freely you have received; now freely give!

If an opportunity to lay hands on someone occurs, go for it—regardless of whether you feel anything or not. You'll be in the miracle ministry, too!

Chapter Sixteen

Spare Parts Department

by Frances

God has a warehouse of spare parts! God made you, and He is smarter than General Motors. General Motors has spare parts for all of their automobiles. God has new parts for you, too.

A girl heard me say one time that God has a warehouse of spare parts and she thought, "I'm not sure I believe that." She had rheumatic fever when she was a young girl, and it left her with a bad heart. That was twenty-two years ago, and so she said, "God, would You just let me see a heavenly warehouse so I know that You really have got spare parts?"

If each of us were to figure in our own minds what the warehouse looked like, we would all think of something different as to what the spare parts department in heaven looks like. Maybe if you're a mechanic you would see shelves like you do in an auto parts store. Little parts would be in all these little different places. I always thought about the spare parts department in heaven as being like a freezer of a meat cooler in a grocery store, where they have these big hooks hanging up with beef carcasses hanging on them. I could see hearts hanging up there and all kinds of spare parts. But this girl said, "God, let me see what a warehouse of spare parts is."

Later, in amazement, she said, "I still don't know if it was a dream or a vision or what it was, but suddenly I saw a river of water, clear as crystal, flowing out of the throne room of God. It was so cold and it was so clear and there were some things just bouncing up and down all over. I looked a little closer, and they were hearts! All hearts, and they were in this cold, clear water!" She was fascinated watching all these hearts go by, and suddenly one appeared that had the name Susan on it. She said, "I'll take it!" And as she grabbed for the heart with the name Susan on it, she was instantly healed by the power of God!

It's like a retread on a car tire. You see them all over the highways. Get a new part—not a retread. Charles and I never ask for a repair job on people. If you've got something that's worn out, we always ask for a new one. I got an interesting fax when I was down in Mexico on my birthday. It was from the president of Channel 40 TV station in Pittsburgh. He said, "Frances, since your heart is less than twenty-five years old, your thyroid is thirty years old, your pancreas is twelve years old, and your blood system is eight, how much of the original Frances Hunter is there left to wish happy birthday?" Hallelujah!

All of the new parts God has given to me have been confirmed by doctors before and after the new parts have been given to me.

I said to Charles, "I'd have a difficult time dying, because all my parts are different ages." Some are very young, some are slightly old, and some are the original ones. Don't hesitate to ask God for a new part, because He has a sufficient supply for everyone!

The Word of God tells us that we can call into being those things that are not as though they were, and we have seen some incredible things happen as we have called into being new hearts, new livers, new stomachs, and many other parts. Remember when you're praying for the sick that you have absolutely nothing to lose, because you can't do anything to make them worse. All you can do is leave them in an improved or healed condition.

Over the years many, many people have come up to us and have said something similar to this: "You laid hands on me fifteen years ago for a new heart. I received a new heart and have never had a problem from that day to this!"

These are not the types of healings that you can tell about instantly, because there's no way we can look on the inside of you to see whether or not you have received a new heart, a new liver, or any other organ. But time will tell, and it's such a delight to us to have people come up and say, as someone recently did, "You laid hands on me twenty-six years ago for a new liver. I was dying of cancer, and my liver was swollen and distended, but you laid hands on me. Within two months the cancer had totally disappeared, and the liver was absolutely normal."

What rejoicing there was in my heart because this also proves that God's healings last. Many people are inclined to believe that people just get "hyped up" in services and that the healings will disappear as soon as they get home. This is totally untrue because God's healings will last unless we let doubt or unbelief bring the same thing back on us. They will stand up under an X ray or blood test!

Try calling into being some new parts that you may need and see what happens. You will be delighted, especially with the first doctor's diagnosis that says, "I don't understand what happened, but you have a new heart!"

Remember, if Charles and Frances can do it, you can do it too! That means calling into being new parts in the name of Jesus.

Use the command: "In Jesus' name, I command a creative miracle; I call into being the things (name the part you need) that are not as though they are." (See Romans 4:17.)

Chapter Seventeen

It Works in Every Nation

by Frances

It doesn't matter what language you speak, whether it's English, Spanish, Russian, Korean, or any other language in the world; the Word of God works wherever you are. It doesn't just work in sections; it works all the way, whether you're talking about healing and health, prosperity, or peace of mind and heart. The Word of God works through any language in the world!

On January 1, 1996, I received a phone call from Acapulco, Mexico. The caller said, "Frances, how would you like to celebrate your eightieth birthday with a Healing Explosion in Acapulco?" The Holy

Spirit quickened me, and my answer immediately came back, "Yes, I would love to celebrate my birthday that way!" That was the start of one of the most incredible Healing Explosions we have ever had in our entire lives. The first training session was a great surprise, because they had to take it outdoors to an amphitheater to accommodate the large crowd. Instead of a crowd between 800 and 900, they had over 2,400 at the first training session. That's a lot of learning!

When the night came for the actual Healing Explosion, the faith of the people had risen so high because of the miracles they had seen happen during the training sessions. Believing what we said was true—"If Charles and Frances can do it, you can do it too"—they attacked the sicknesses with an aggressiveness that we had never seen up until that time.

Often people ask us, "How do you stay so excited all the time about Jesus?" There is only one reason: Christianity is not a religion; it is a way of life that you live twenty-four hours of every day.

The last words of Jesus on earth were, "Preach the Gospel to every creature." (See Mark 16:15–18, the Great Commission.) That's the reason Jesus came to earth—to save the lost!

Then Jesus gave us the rest of our work assign-ment—to do miracles, including healing the sick.

Remember always that Christ in you is the only hope of glory! Start believing that He is actually living inside of you and that when you stretch forth your hand, it's the hand of Jesus being laid on the sick. The more this becomes a living reality in our lives, the more we can accomplish for the kingdom of God, regardless of where we live or what language we speak. We don't believe the people in Acapulco will ever be the same again!

Chapter Eighteen

As You Are Going...

by Frances

When Jesus told us to go, He meant "as you are going"—going about your daily business, at work, in school, at the park, at the shopping center, before and after church, in the restaurant, at the health club, at prayer meetings, at coffee or lunch breaks, or wherever your daily life takes you. We should be fulfilling the Great Commission on a continual daily basis.

Walk, run, or fly with us through a few of the events of our normal daily walk with Jesus!

Flying to a meeting one day, the man sitting next to us stood up. We noticed a special back pillow in his seat. To us that was a signal for a miracle. When he returned, we questioned him about his back.

He was a salesman who traveled overseas as well as in the United States. He said the pain was so excruciating that he didn't believe he would be able to make it to Korea the next week.

As we were getting off the plane in the next city, we asked him, "Would you like to go to the lobby and let us pray for your back to be healed?" When you're hurting badly enough, you will never resist such an offer. We told him he had nothing to lose.

He was in such severe pain as he hobbled to the lobby that he was almost in tears. He didn't want to sit down in public, so we put him behind the ticket counter wall.

His back was so out of line, we discovered, that one leg was two inches shorter than the other. When it grew out, he jumped up, bent over, twisted his back, and then heard, "Final boarding call!" He ran down the ramp as fast as he could, yelling, "I have no more pain!"

Another healing occurred on a recent trip when we stopped at the only restaurant open at that hour of the night. After seating us at a dirty, oil-cloth-covered table, the waitress gave us the menus. Charles noticed something. He said to the waitress, "My wife has a wonderful ministry for pregnant women. Would you like for her to pray for you?"

The young woman burst into laughter and said, "Pray?" and continued laughing.

I immediately sensed a wonderful "as we were going" opportunity. So, grabbing her left hand, I laid my hand on her tummy and said, "Father, I thank You for this beautiful baby. Thank You that we don't believe in abortion." Before I said another word, she burst into tears. I knew she had considered abortion. I asked her whether she was married because there was no ring on her finger. She stumbled for words and finally came out with a very weak, "Yes."

I said, "You need Jesus, honey. Pray this prayer after me."

She prayed, and when we finished, I asked her, "Where is Jesus right now?"

She said, "In my heart!" The girl we left behind was not the same girl we met when we came in. She was a new creature!

Use every opportunity for God to do miracles through Jesus in you—as you are going!

Chapter Nineteen

Don't Forget

by Charles and Frances

1. Ask the person to whom you are ministering what his problem is. What does his doctor say is wrong?

2. It is not important to know all the medical details of an illness to be able to minister healing. It is important to know what the problem is, and to address the problem itself, rather than the symptoms. Above all, remember to be practical, which means to listen carefully to what the person is saying so that you minister healing to the specific problem.

3. When you ask someone what his disease is, say, "That's easy" after his answer, regardless of how difficult his condition may sound. Remember the most fatal disease is "easy" when God steps in. We have discovered that this reply gives hope to the one to

whom you are ministering, and also increases your faith to hear yourself tell someone that his problem is "easy."

4. Once you have ministered healing, have the person put his faith into action. If his back was hurting, have him bend his back. If the problem was in his elbow, have him bend the elbow. If the problem was arthritis in the shoulder or knees, have him either swing the arm or move the leg and knee area.

5. Make sure the person says, "Thank You, Jesus!" Thanksgiving to Him can complete an incomplete healing.

6. Learn to look for the ones who are healed. If you look for the ones who are not healed, your faith will tend to waver; so continue looking only for the ones who are healed, and watch the percentage grow!

7. People will often say, "It still hurts," and when you ask them how much of the pain is gone, they will say, "Ninety-five percent, but there's still a little bit left." Encourage them to thank God for the 95 percent that's gone, because when they do, often the last 5 percent will be manifested. We have also discovered that if they emphasize the negative, the 95 percent will drop to 90 percent and will continue to go down. Thanking Jesus is one of the best ways to get a healing completed! And by the same token, being negative can cause the 5 percent of the pain to increase to 10 percent and then to 15 percent, and so on, until an individual has all the pain back and has totally lost his healing.

8. Look for the absence of pain, not the pain! Look for the healing, not the sickness!

9. You are not a doctor, so don't try to practice medicine. Do not prescribe medication or recommend that people go off of their medication.

10. Do not make a diagnosis. Let the individual to whom you are ministering tell you what his problem and symptoms are.

11. Whenever you cast out a spirit, do it "in the name of Jesus and by the power of God's Holy Spirit."

12. Remember, there are two things necessary for healings to be accomplished: the name of Jesus (say it over and over again; you can't say it too much!) and the power of God's Holy Spirit.

13. If one thing doesn't work, ask God what to do. Keep trying different things and be persistent.

14. If after ministering to the individual the best you know how, there are still no visible results, then encourage that person to believe the healing has started because the healing power of God has gone into him. It's amazing how many discover later that they were healed.

15. Never do anything half-heartedly for the Lord.

16. When in doubt, cast it out!

17. When in doubt, grow it out!

18. After you have ministered healing to more than one thing, you will find it helpful to go through "the arm

thing" and "the leg thing" again after ministering in other areas.

19. Before you lay hands on a person, be particularly cautious that you have someone standing behind him to catch him if he goes under the power. Hold him by the shoulders if there is no catcher available. If a person does not fall under the power, don't be concerned. Some do, and some do not! But people get healed either way!

20. Remember, you are not a physician, a chiropractor, or an osteopath, and are not making adjustments, but applying the supernatural power of God.

21. Walk in boldness. Don't let fear stop you. Speak with authority. That doesn't mean speak loudly, but when you mean what you say, say it like you mean it.

22. A force field of power comes out of you. The closer you are to the person, the more power he will feel and receive. Stand close but in good taste.

23. Concentrate on one of his problems at a time when you minister healing; don't minister to all the physical problems in the same sentence. Do one at a time. Check to see how the first condition is progressing before going on with the next. Start with something he can quickly know it is healed, if possible, such as a pain or discomfort that can be easily identified. "Growing out arms or legs," "the pelvic thing," or "the neck thing" is almost always a good way to start.

24. Healing the sick takes persistence and practice. Everyone to whom you minister at first may not necessarily be healed, but Jesus promised that we would do the same things He did, and even greater things. He healed all who came to Him for healing. We believe that eventually all who come to the Spirit-filled believing body of Christ for healing will be healed. The key is to never stop obeying the Great Commission Jesus gave us in Mark 16:15–18.

25. We can call into being those things which are not as though they are. (See Romans 4:17.) God has a whole warehouse of spare parts. A new tire is better than a retread. Did you ever notice the retreads that "blow" on the highway and have pieces scattered all over the place? Go for a new part. Charles says that I have more new parts than I have originals!

26. Don't let people lose their healing through doubt and unbelief. Stay with them until they actually know that they are healed. The devil comes to steal their healing, so don't let him. Make sure they continue to praise God.

27. Don't sit on the back burner waiting for God to call you. He has already called you according to Mark 16:15–18, and He told you what to do. He said, *"These signs will follow those who believe:...they will lay hands on the sick, and they will recover"* (verses 17–18). Beloved, God is doing a new thing. God's message for the hour is for us, all of us, as believers, to go out and lay hands on the sick. Then God will do His part, and they will recover.

28. When Jesus was ministering here on earth, He did not work up emotions or give long complicated prayers. He simply spoke healing into the person. If you are baptized with the Holy Spirit, then that same power that raised Jesus from the dead flows out of you. It is God's power that touches a person's body, and it is His power that does the healing. When you lay hands on people in Jesus' name, the healing virtue of God flows from the Spirit of God within you to those to whom you are ministering.

29. Since you are filled with the Holy Spirit, and He is the Anointed One, then His anointing power is always in you. So keep in mind that the anointing is not something that comes and goes periodically, but He remains within you.

30. At times the question comes up, Can you get people healed if they have doubt and unbelief? The Bible says that signs will follow those who believe. We also know that Jesus healed so that people would believe. It is true that unbelief can stop healing, yet often those who are watching when someone gets healed are the first to repent and receive Jesus as Savior.

31. Never forget to use wisdom, common sense, good judgment, and discretion. In other words, don't be a "flake."

32. Be careful not to minister on a long-term basis together with someone of the opposite sex, unless it is your wife or husband. As soon as possible find a partner who is the same sex as you are, especially

when you are going out to minister in the community.

33. If someone needs healing in a private part of his body, have him put his hand over or near the area, then place your hand on top of his. Be discreet in all you do, for you represent Jesus.

34. Don't allow yourself to become discouraged. The devil loves to come in on the situation and try to cause your faith to go right out your feet. You may find yourself facing a difficult disease the first time you step out. Don't let it throw you. Just remember this: if you are dead to self, then you won't worry about what people say. Just do your best, asking the Holy Spirit to lead you and to speak to you.

35. When ministering to someone who has a sore or an open cut or a discharge, do not place your hand directly on the affected area. Instead, have the person place his hand near or over the area; then place your hand on top of his to minister. Of course God's power can prevent spreading disease, but we are in the world and are subject to natural laws of God. After ministering, be sure to wash your hands thoroughly. This is just good common hygiene.

36. When ministering to anyone, please find out if he is saved. If he is not, minister salvation.

37. Always determine if the person to whom you are ministering has received the baptism with the Holy Spirit and speaks in tongues. If not, then minister to him.

38. Be bold!

39. Having done all, stand! (See Ephesians 6:13.)

Chapter Twenty

Diseases from A to Z

Listed in this chapter, in alphabetical order, are many common diseases for which you will be ministering healing and deliverance. Some of these will require the same approach as others, so in our listing, we will simply state what to do. The "how to do it" is covered either in the book *How to Heal the Sick,* in this book, or in the video and audio tapes entitled *How to Heal the Sick.*

THE NAME OF JESUS

The name of Jesus is above every other name. You cannot repeat this too much or too often. Jesus gave us the authority to cast out devils and to minister healing to whatever disease people have. When you speak "in the name of Jesus" or "in Jesus' name," that means you are ministering by the authority Jesus has given to you, a believer.

Jesus gave us the responsibility to use that power and authority to do His works on earth and to destroy the works of the devil.

Remember, whatever we bind on earth is bound in heaven, and whatever we loose on earth is loosed in heaven.

Common sense and basic knowledge may lead you to minister in greater detail than shown herein. Be alert to comments and answers given by the one to whom you are ministering.

The Holy Spirit will lead you more specifically as you minister to a person, learning his needs. Let your very soul reach out in compassion to meet his needs, whatever the disease.

SUGGESTED SALVATION PRAYER

Father, in the name of Jesus, I ask You to forgive all of my sins. Jesus, come into my heart and live in me. Thank You, Jesus, for coming into my heart. Thank You that all my sins are forgiven and that I have been born again.

TO CAST OUT A SPIRIT

Say, "Devil (or Satan), I bind you in the name of Jesus, and by the power of God's Holy Spirit. You foul spirit of _____, come out in the name of Jesus!

For incurable diseases, don't forget to to command the electrical and chemical frequencies in every cell to be in harmony and in balance, in Jesus' name!

IMMUNE SYSTEM

Most diseases start when the immune system is destroyed or low. The immune system is the gatekeeper, the system that admits sickness, or the deficiency that opens the door for sickness, into the body.

It is good to add this command wherever applicable: "We command your immune system to be healed and alert to halt diseases and germs from inflicting this body, in Jesus' name."

HOW TO MINISTER TO VARIOUS DISEASES

A

ABUSE
Remember, it is not the child's fault that the abuse occurred, nor is abuse limited to children.

How to Minister:
1. Lay hands on their heads, asking God to erase the memories.
2. Speak the peace of God upon them.

ACNE, SEVERE

Multiple skin infections (pimples, sores), usually caused by overactivity of the sebaceous (oil) glands of the skin.

How to Minister:

1. Rebuke (or curse) the infection and command it to go.
2. Cast out the spirit of inheritance.
3. Lay hands on the head, commanding the skin pores to open and the sebaceous glands to drain normally.
4. Command the bulbs that manufacture skin cells to manufacture normal functioning skin.

ADDICTION (ALCOHOL, CIGARETTE, OR DRUG)

Physical and psychological dependence on a substance, e.g., alcohol, nicotine in cigarettes, or drugs (e.g., tranquilizers, cocaine, marijuana, heroin, etc.).

How to Minister:

1. Ask the person if he wants to be set free.
2. Ask him if he is saved.
3. Lead the person in the prayer of salvation.
4. Bind and cast out the spirit of alcohol, drug, and/or tobacco addiction.
5. Command the body to be healed and the desire for the drugs, tobacco, and/or alcohol to be gone.

ADDISON'S DISEASE

Failure of the adrenal glands to produce necessary adrenal hormones. See also Cushing's Syndrome.

How to Minister:

1. Command a creative miracle—a new pair of adrenal glands.
2. Command the hormone levels to be normal.

ADENOIDS, SWOLLEN

How to Minister:
1. Place hand on the nose/throat area, commanding the adenoids to shrink and become normal.
2. Do "TNT."

ADHESIONS

See Scar Tissue.

ADRENAL GLAND

An endocrine gland located adjacent to the kidneys. Produces hormones and "flight" or "fight" energy necessary to the body.

See also chapter 12, "The Spine."

How to Minister:
1. "Grow out the arms" and lay hands over the kidneys, commanding the adrenal glands to function properly.
2. Ask if the person has any unforgiveness, explaining that anger or other negative emotions cause the adrenal glands to over-secrete adrenalin, which can contribute to arthritis, blood pressure, or other problems.

AGORAPHOBIA (PANIC ATTACKS)

Severe anxiety causing a fear of going into open places or public areas.

How to Minister:
1. Cast out the spirits of fear and anxiety.
2. Speak the peace of God into the person's heart.
3. Recommend that he fill his mind with the Word of God.
4. Minister salvation and the baptism with the Holy Spirit if applicable.

AIDS

See chapter 11, "When Ministering Healing."

ALLERGIES

Body's negative reaction to a foreign substance. Includes hay fever, drug reactions, food allergies, etc.

See also Asthma.

How to Minister:

1. Cast out the spirits of inheritance and allergy.
2. Lay hands on the head, commanding the immune system to return to normal, and all the tissues and organs to be healed and function normally.
3. Do "TTT."

ALZHEIMER'S DISEASE

A disease of unknown cause that results in deterioration of the brain with memory and reasoning loss.

How to Minister:

1. Cast out the spirits of Alzheimer's disease and inheritance.
2. Speak a creative miracle and command a new brain.

AMBLYOPIA

See Eyes.

AMYOTROPIC LATERAL SCLEROSIS, ALS

Also known as Lou Gehrig's disease. A degeneration of the nerves of the spinal cord with progressive weakness. Medically irreversible.

How to Minister:

1. Bind and cast out the spirit of ALS.
2. Do "TTT," commanding a creative miracle for all new nerves in the spinal cord and body.

ANEMIA

A reduction below normal of red blood cells.

How to Minister:

1. Command the bone marrow to be healed and to manufacture normal amounts of healthy red blood cells.

ANEMIA, PERNICIOUS

Low blood count caused by a failure to absorb vitamin B-12 from the G.I. (gastrointestinal) tract.

How to Minister:
1. Command the intestinal tract to be healed and to properly absorb and utilize vitamin B-12.
2. Command the bone marrow to produce rich, healthy red blood cells.

ANEURYSM

A condition where the artery wall is thinned and stretched out; possibility of rupture exists. Can occur anywhere in the body.

How to Minister:
1. Lay hands on the affected area, commanding a creative miracle—new arteries with good strong walls.
2. Command restoration of normal blood flow.

ANOREXIA NERVOSA

An eating disorder where the person is practically starving himself, usually emotionally based.

How to Minister:
1. Bind and cast out the spirits of rejection and anorexia.
2. Speak peace and self-confidence to the person.
3. Ask if he is saved—have him repeat the prayer of salvation.
4. Explain that our bodies are God's holy temple and we must not do anything to injure ourselves, e.g., not eating, self-induced vomiting, etc.
5. Command the "appestat" (the appetite control center in the brain) to be reset for a normal appetite.

"Appestat"

The brain's control center for the appetite (or desire for food).
See chapter 13, "The 'Appestat.'"

How to Minister:

1. Lay hands on the front and back of the head, commanding the "appestat" to be healed.
2. Command the metabolism to function normally and the person's weight to be within healthy boundaries.

Arches

See Feet.

Arms and Hands

Numbness, tingling, and pain usually caused by a neck problem.

How to Minister:

1. "Grow out the arms."
2. Do "TNT," commanding the vertebrae and discs to align and the nerves to be restored to normal structure and function.
3. Minister healing to other causes.

Arteriosclerosis

Hardening of the arteries caused by deposits of cholesterol inside the arteries (blood vessels).

How to Minister:

1. Do "TNT."
2. Speak a divine "roto-rooter" of God's power to completely clean out all the arteries of all cholesterol plaques.

ARTHRITIS

A painful inflammation of the joints.
See the chapter 12, "The Spine."

How to Minister:
1. Bind and cast out the spirit of arthritis.
2. Command the inflammation to be healed and pain to go.
3. Do "TNT" and "TPT."
4. Mention that most arthritis stems from harbored anger and resentment or unforgiveness. Pray a prayer of forgiveness.

ASTHMA

Condition in the lungs causing wheezing and shortness of breath. Often runs in families and is often associated with allergies.

How to Minister:
1. Cast out the spirit of asthma.
2. Do "TNT."
3. "Grow out the arms."
4. Speak the peace of God into the person's life.

ASTIGMATISM

See Eyes.

AUTISM OR ATTENTION DEFICIT DISORDER (A.D.D.)

Usually caused by a brain problem.
See chapter 11, "When Ministering Healing."

How to Minister:
1. Use extreme gentleness and a quiet attitude; hold the person if possible.
2. Speaking softly but firmly, bind and cast out the spirit of autism.
3. While touching the person, command a new brain and the total restoration of nervous system.
4. Speak the peace of God into the heart and soul.

B

BACK PROBLEMS

How to Minister:

1. Determine what to do by finding out what is wrong (e.g., what is the doctor's diagnosis? What do you know is wrong specifically? Do you have pain? Were you in an accident? Have you had surgery?).
2. Do "TNT." For healing above the waist, "Grow out the arms." For healing below the waist, "Grow out legs" and do "TPT."
3. Do any or all of these as needed and repeat if necessary.
4. Command the discs, vertebrae, muscles, ligaments, and tendons to be healed and adjusted. Be specific in making the command to the extent you know what is wrong.

Disc Problems

Commonly called "slipped disc." Disc (or cushion) between two vertebrae (bones in your back) has either deteriorated or is bulging out, pressing on a nerve and causing discomfort and pain.

How to Minister:

1. Do "TTT" (or minister as explained above), commanding the disc to be restored and be healed, recreated if necessary; all pressure on the nerves to be released.
2. Command the vertebrae to be healed, rotated back into place, bones to come together if fractured, ribs be healed and go back into place. Deal with each specific back problem one at a time if you have enough information. Use common sense. Test the person's healing. Have him put his faith into action.

BALANCE, LOSS OF

How to Minister:
1. Ask what the person's doctor says has caused the problem.
2. Rebuke the cause (e.g., infection, disease, etc.) of the loss of balance.
3. Do "TNT" and "grow out the arms," commanding the balance center in the inner ear to be healed and the temporal bones to rotate back into position.

Dizziness or Vertigo

Dizziness is one of the most common neurological symptoms encountered in medical practice. The most common form of dizziness is known as vertigo. This term describes a sensation of motion when there is no motion, or an exaggerated sense of motion in response to certain body movements.

Vertigo and dizziness are symptoms linked to a variety of inner ear disturbances and other systemic illness. The sensation of dizziness is frequently accompanied by other symptoms, such as unsteadiness, lightheadedness, anxiety, etc.

How to Minister:
1. Command the electrical and chemical frequencies in every cell of the inner ear and brain to be in harmony and in balance and to digest all impaired cells; command normal balance to return.
2. Command the normal flow of oxygen to flow to the brain.

BALDNESS

Inability to grow normal amounts of hair on the head.

How to Minister:
1. Command healing to the hair follicles.
2. Command the hair to be restored to normal growth.

BARRENNESS

See Infertility.

BED-WETTING

Almost always will have a short leg.

How to Minister:

1. "Grow out the legs" and do "TPT," commanding the vertebrae in the lower back to be adjusted, the nerves to the bladder to be released, the bladder to be healed and function properly.
2. Speak blessings on the child. We normally also whisper a prayer in his ear, asking God to station an angel with him to awaken him if he needs to go to the bathroom at night, so he need not be afraid.

BELL'S PALSY

Damage to the nerve on the side of the face; may be due to a virus infection; normally causes severe pain and paralysis of the facial muscles with a drooping appearance.

How to Minister:

1. Cast out the spirit causing Bell's palsy.
2. Command the pain to go.
3. Lay hands gently on the face, commanding the nerves to be regenerated and restored to perfect function.

BIRTH (PRAYER FOR EASY DELIVERY)

How to Minister:

1. Ask Jesus to bless the baby in the womb with the power of the Holy Spirit and dedicate the child to God.
2. Ask God to oil the birth canal with the oil of the Holy Spirit and let the baby slide painlessly out within three hours after the mother reaches the hospital.

BLADDER PROBLEMS

Lack of Control
Usually caused by damage to structures or nerves.

How to Minister:
1. Command the bladder and nerve tissues to be healed and restored to normal function.
2. "Grow out the legs."
3. Do "TPT."

Infections
May be caused by abnormal anatomy, especially if frequent infections are occuring.

How to Minister:
1. Rebuke the infection.
2. Do "TPT" and "grow out the legs," commanding the bladder and all the tissues and nerves to be restored to normal structure and function.

BLINDNESS
See Eyes.

BLOOD PRESSURE PROBLEMS
Caused by numerous dysfunctions of the body organs. Ask if the doctor has diagnosed any possible underlying causes (e.g., diabetes, arteriosclerosis, kidney problems, heart disease, etc.).

How to Minister:
1. Command the heart to be healed, the arteries and vessels to be opened and function normally with proper elasticity. Include other organs if a diagnosis was made involving them also.
2. Do "TNT" and "grow out the arms," commanding the muscles and nerves to be normal and allow blood to flow properly.

BOWED LEGS

Knees swing outward, giving person a "cowboy" look.

How to Minister:

Do "TPT" and "grow out the legs," commanding the legs to straighten.

BRAIN DAMAGE

How to Minister:

1. If caused by a stroke, command the spirit of death of the brain cells to come out.
2. Lay hands on the head, commanding a creative miracle—a new brain (brain tissue is not regenerated by the body).
3. Command all the nerves to function normally and any memory loss to be restored.

BROKEN BONES

How to Minister:

1. Lay hands on the affected area, commanding the affected bones to come together in normal alignment and strength and be healed.
2. Command all muscles, tendons, nerves, and ligaments to line up with the healed bones and strengthen the area previously damaged.

BRONCHITIS

Irritation and inflammation of the bronchial tubes (connecting the nose to the lungs).

How to Minister:

1. Rebuke the infection.
2. Lay hands on the upper chest and throat, commanding the tissues in the bronchial tubes and lungs to be healed and function normally.

BULIMIA

A constant, excessive, insatiable appetite, and often induced vomiting and eating in a repeated cycle.

See chapter 13, "The 'Appestat.'"

How to Minister:

1. Cast out the spirits of bulimia, rejection and anxiety.
2. Do "TNT," commanding the "appestat" to be readjusted to normal.
3. Speak peace, self-confidence, and love to the person's spirit and soul.

BUNION

See Feet.

BURSITIS

Inflammation of fluid-filled sacs (bursas) that facilitate tendon/muscle movement over bones.

How to Minister:

1. Cast out the spirit of bursitis.
2. Touch the affected area and command all inflammation and pain to go, all tissues to be healed, and normal fluid be produced for painless movement of the joints.

C

CANCER

A tumor that grows progressively through the body. Includes leukemia, lymphoma, and other malignant tumors.

See Chapter 7, "Electrical and Chemical Frequencies."

How to Minister:

1. Bind and cast out the spirit of cancer.
2. Curse the seed, root, and cells of the cancer.
3. Lay hands on the affected area, commanding every cancer cell in the body to die.
4. Command the bone marrow to produce pure, healthy blood.
5. Command healing to all organs and tissues affected and restoration of parts where necessary.
6. Command the body's defensive "killer" cells to multiply and attack all cancer cells.

CANDIDA

A fungal (yeast) infection that affects the mucous membranes of the body; generally cause of vaginal infections; aggravated by sugar intake; cause of thrush (a form of candida) in children.

How to Minister:

1. Rebuke the infection.
2 Command the body's systems to be restored to normal function.
3. "Grow out the legs" and do "TPT," commanding nerves and muscles to be relaxed and normal.

CARPAL TUNNEL SYNDROME

A nerve is compressed inside the wrist (carpal tunnel), leading to pain and weakness in the hand.

How to Minister:

1. Lay hands on the wrist area and command the tissues, tendons, and ligaments in the wrist to be healed and relaxed.
2. Command the "tunnel" to open up and pressure on the nerve to be released, to be healed and to function normally.
3. "Grow out the arms" and do "TNT," commanding normal circulation and strength to be restored.

CATARACTS

See chapter "Eye Healings."

CEREBRAL PALSY

How to Minister:

1. Cast out the spirit of cerebral palsy.
2. Speak a new brain into body.
3. Do "TTT," activating the communication from the brain to the other body parts, commanding the muscles, tendons, and nerves to function properly.

CHOLESTEROL, HIGH

Too much fat in diet.

How to Minister:

1. Command the cholesterol level to return to normal and the body to retain only the necessary amounts.
2. Lay hands on the person's head, commanding all potentially damaged parts of the body (e.g., arteries, heart, etc.) to become normal.

CIGARETTES

See Addictions.

CLEFT PALATE

An undeveloped roof of the mouth.

How to Minister:
1. Cast out the spirit of inheritance.
2. Lay hands on the mouth, commanding a creative miracle; all the tissues and structures to be normal.

COLD SORES

See Herpes.

COLDS

See Influenza.

COLITIS

How to Minister:
1. Do "TPT" and "grow out legs," commanding the nerves controlling the colon to be loosed.
2. Command the colon to be healed.

COMA

Unconsciousness caused by disease or severe trauma.

How to Minister:
1. Cast out the spirit of death of brain cells.
2. Lay hands on the head, commanding the brain to be healed; command a creative miracle to any damaged brain tissue (brain tissue will not regenerate on its own).
3. Command the body and all its organs to operate normally and consciousness to return.
4. Speak to the person's soul—his soul is not in a coma. Lead him to Jesus if he is not saved. Even though he cannot say the prayer, his soul can respond.

CONSTIPATION

Usually caused by dietary problems.

How to Minister:

Do "TPT" and "grow out the legs," commanding the colon to function normally.

CORNS

See Feet.

CROHN'S DISEASE

Chronic inflammation of the mucous membranes of the intestinal tract.

How to Minister:

1. Cast out the spirit of Crohn's disease.
2. Rebuke the infection.
3. "Grow out the legs" and do "TPT," commanding the bowel tissue to be healed and function normally.

CUSHING'S SYNDROME

Overactivity of the adrenal glands.

How to Minister:

1. Cast out the Cushing's Syndrome spirit.
2. Lay hands on the kidney area of the back, commanding the adrenal glands to function properly.

CYSTIC DISEASE

Condition affecting women, usually near or at menopause; characterized by rapid development of cysts in a breast. Also called fibrocystic disease or cystic mastitis.

How to Minister:

1. Cast out the spirit of fibrocystic disease.
2. Lay hands on chest, commanding all the cysts to dissolve and disappear, all the cells and tissues of the breast to be healed and normal, and a creative miracle for any damaged parts.

CYSTIC FIBROSIS

An inherited disease leading to chronic lung disease; most commonly found only in children because usual lifespan of these people is very short; also affects the pancreas and liver.

How to Minister:

1. Bind and cast out the spirits of inheritance and cystic fibrosis.
2. Lay hands on the area of the pancreas and liver, commanding the glands of the body to secrete normally.
3. Command the lungs, pancreas, and liver to be healed and function normally.

D

DEAF-MUTE

Person who can neither hear nor speak.

How to Minister:

1. Cast out the deaf and dumb spirit.
2. Continue instructions as for Deafness.
3. Test both hearing and speaking.

DEAFNESS

May be caused by a deaf spirit attaching itself to the body, an inherited spirit, nerve failure, punctured or damaged eardrum. Determine by inquiry, if possible, the cause of the deafness and the percent of hearing loss.

See Chapter 7, "Electrical and Chemical Frequencies."

How to Minister:
1. Cast out the spirit of deafness.
2. Put your fingers gently in the person's ears and command the deafness to go and hearing to be restored.
3. Grow out their arms.
4. Command a new eardrum and bone structures, if needed.
5. Do "TNT," commanding the nerves and muscles to relax, releasing the nerves to the ears, and allowing the blood to flow into the ears, and commanding the hairlike nerves to the inner ear to grow.
6. Place the hands on the sides of the skull and command the temporal bones to rotate back into position. Test the person's hearing and repeat the above if necessary.

DEPRESSION

See Mental Illness.

DERMATITIS

Inflammation of the skin.

How to Minister:
1. Rebuke the infection and itching.
2. Command cells that manufacture skin to create new and healthy tissue.

DETATCHED RETINA

See Eyes.

DIABETES

Lack of insulin production by pancreas.

See also Hypoglycemia.

How to Minister:
1. Cast out the spirits of inheritance and diabetes.
2. Command a new pancreas into the body.
3. Command any damaged body parts (from excess sugar) to be healed and made whole.

DIARRHEA
1. Do "TTT."
2. Command digestive system to be healed, and rebuke infection.

DISC DISEASE

See Back Problems.

DIVERTICULOSIS/DIVERTICULISIS

Outpouchings (small herniated sacs) of the mucous membrane of the bowel through the muscular wall.

See also Crohn's Disease.

How to Minister:
1. Do "TPT," commanding the sacs to disappear and the bowel wall to return to normal strength and function.
2. Command infection to go and tissues to be totally healed.

DOWAGER'S HUMP

See Osteoporosis.

Down's Syndrome

How to Minister:
1. Bind and cast out the spirit of Down's Syndrome.
2. Lay hands on the person's head, and command a new brain.
3. Command the cells to revert to the correct number of chromosomes, and for the extra chromosome to go.
4. Command the body to be healed and function normally.
5. Command the facial features to be normal.

Drowning

Excessive fluid into the lungs.

How to Minister:
1. Bind and cast out the spirit of death.
2. Command the water to come out of the lungs.
3. Command life to reenter the body.
4. Command the brain and body to function normally and be totally healed.

Dyslexia

Impairment of the ability to read.

How to Minister:
1. Command the nerves of the eyes to function normally and to send proper messages to the brain.
2. Command the brain to interpret signals received and impart understanding to the person.

E

EARS

Tinnitus

Abnormal ringing, roaring, or hissing in the ears.

How to Minister:
1. Cast out the spirit of tinnitus.
2. Do "TNT."
3. Command the blood to flow through the ear canal.

Fungus or Infection

How to Minister:
1. Rebuke the fungus or infection.
2. Do "TNT" and command the blood to flow into the ears and remove impurities.

Meniere's Disease

How to Minister:
1. Cast out spirit of Meniere's Disease.
2. Command ears to be healed and balance restored.

ECZEMA

Disease of the skin.

How to Minister:
1. Cast out the spirit of eczema.
2. Command the inflammation to go. Curse the infirmity.
3. Command the cells that manufacture skin to replace the damaged tissues, and the skin to return to normal structure, function, and texture.

EDEMA

Abnormal collection of fluid in the body. Also called dropsy.

How to Minister:
1. Command healing for any underlying disease.
2. Command that the involved organs or tissues be healed and function normally.
3. Command a divine diuretic (cause the fluid to pass through the body).

EMPHYSEMA

Lung disease; the inability to breathe properly.

How to Minister:
1. Minister deliverance from smoking, if necessary.
2. Minister salvation and baptism of the Holy Spirit, if needed.
3. "Grow out the arms," commanding a creative miracle—a new set of lungs with healthy lung tissue to function properly.
4. Command other damaged body tissue to become normal.

ENCEPHALITIS

Inflammation of the brain. Usually caused by a viral infection.

How to Minister:
1. Rebuke the infection.
2. Command the swelling to go and the brain to be healed, restored, and function normally.
3. Do "TNT," commanding the blood to flow normally into the brain.

ENDOMETRIOSIS

Tumor/tissue in female organs. Pain with the menstrual period.

How to Minister:
1. Do "TPT," commanding the female organs to function normally.
2. "Grow out the legs."
3. Command the extra tissue to dissolve and disappear.

EPILEPSY

Brain problem; seizures.

How to Minister:

1. Cast out the spirit of epilepsy. (Jesus did!)
2. Do "TNT."

EYES

See chapter 14, "Eye Healings."

Astigmatism

Abnormal shape of the eye.

How to Minister:

1. Command all parts of the eye to be healed and return to normal shape.
2. Do "TNT."

Blindness

Vision damage. Determine, if you can, how much the person can see before and after ministering.

How to Minister:

1. If the cause is known, address it specifically (e.g., glaucoma, cataracts, infection, detached retina, etc.).
2. Bind and cast out the spirit of blindness.
3. Command healing to the eyes and perfect sight to be restored.
4. Do "TNT."
5. Command a creative miracle to the nerves, eye structures, and brain.

Cataract

A clouding of the lens of the eye.

How to Minister:

1. Lay hands on eyes.
2. Command the blood and fluid to flow through the "onion" layers.

Cross-eyed or Walleyed

Eyes focus inward or eyes focus outward, respectively.

How to Minister:

1. Place your hands over the eyes and command the muscles, ligaments, and tissues to be healed and return to normal strength and length.
2. Command any scar tissue to be removed.

Detached Retina

How to Minister:

1. Lay hands on the eye(s) and command the retina and its nerve endings to reconnect to the eye and be healed.
2. Command the eye to function normally and eyesight to be restored to normal.

Dry Eyes

How to Minister:

1. Command any blockage or abnormality to be gone and healing to take place.
2. Command the glands to produce normal amounts of fluid to keep the eyes healthy.

Farsightedness

Inability to see items up close.

How to Minister:

1. Lay hands on the eyes, commanding the lens, nerves, ligaments, and muscles to be adjusted and work properly.
2. Command perfect sight to be restored.

Floaters or "Webbing"

How to Minister:

1. Lay hands on the eyes, commanding the blood and fluid in the eyes to be restored to normal function and all foreign substances to dissolve and go.
2. Command any scar tissue to be healed.

Glaucoma

Increased pressure within the eyeball.

How to Minister:

1. Command the canals of the eyes to open, and the pressure to normalize and allow fluid to flow normally.
2. Command any disease process or scar tissue to be healed, and eyes to return to normal.

Lazy Eye

How to Minister:

1. Command eye muscles to be of equal length and strength and the nerves to function normally.
2. Command the eye to be healed and vision to be normal.

Macular Degeneration

Retinal deterioration.

How to Minister:

Lay hands over the eyes. Speak a creative miracle and command a new retina.

Nearsightedness

Inability to see far off. Also known as myopia.

How to Minister:

1. Lay hands on the eyes, commanding the lens, nerves, ligaments, and muscles to be adjusted and work properly.
2. Command perfect sight to be restored.

Retinitis Pigmentosa

Shrinking of the retina.

How to Minister:

Lay hands on the eyes, commanding a creative miracle to the eye for a new retina and perfect vision.

F

FEAR

Abnormal fear of normal situations, people, and/or things. Ask what the person fears.

How to Minister:
1. Tell the person that fear is of the devil and perfect love casts out fear.
2. Cast out the spirit of fear.
3. Speak the peace of God into the person, and ask God to spiritually erase the fear and any remembrance of previous episodes.
4. Suggest that the individual read a modern version of the Bible at least one hour a day; memorize 2 Timothy 1:7.
5. Ask God to station a special angel with him.

FEET

Most foot problems are inherited.

How to Minister:
1. Do "TTT"
2. Command the twenty-six bones in each foot to go into proper position and be healed and strong.

Bunions

A swelling in the joint of the big toe.

How to Minister:
1. Cast out the spirit of inheritance.
2. Rebuke the inflammation.
3. Do "TPT" and/or "grow out the legs," commanding the toe and bones to go back into place and the ligaments to strengthen, the foot to be normal.

Callouses and Corns

How to Minister:

Lay hands on the affected area, commanding the corns and callouses to fall off and be replaced by healthy tissue.

Duck Feet

Feet turn excessively outward.

How to Minister:

1. Cast out the spirit of inheritance.
2. Do "TPT" and command the pelvic bones to rotate inward; hips, legs, and feet to return to normal position and be totally healed.

Pigeon Toes

Feet turned inward.

How to Minister:

1. Cast out the spirit of inheritance
2. Do "TPT" and command the pelvic bones to rotate outward and into normal position.

FEMALE PROBLEMS

Any problems with the female reproductive organs of the body. Includes painful menstrual periods, PMS (Premenstrual Syndrome) and prolapsed uterus.

How to Minister:

1. "Grow out the legs" and/or do "TPT" commanding all the tissues, nerves and vessels to function normally and sacrum to rotate into correct position.
2. Command any infection or irritation to go.
3. Command all scar tissue, damaged or destroyed parts to be restored and function properly.
4. Command all hormones to be released within the body in normal amounts and a divine diuretic to rid the body of any excess fluid.

Fibroid Tumors

Benign (not cancerous) tumors of the uterus.
See Chapter 7, "Electrical and Chemical Frequencies."

How to Minister:

1. Cast out the spirit causing the tumor.
2. Command the tumor cells to die and dissolve.
3. "Grow out the legs" and/or do "TPT" commanding the tissues of the reproductive organs be restored to normal function and be totally healed.

FIBROMYALGIA

A mysteriously debilitating syndrome. It is not physically damaging to the body in any way, but is characterized by the constant presence of widespread pain so severe that it is often incapacitating. Other symptoms include, but are not limited to, chronic muscle pain, aching, stiffness, disturbed sleep, depression, and fatigue.

See Chapter 7, "Electrical and Chemical Frequencies."

FISSURE, RECTAL

Crack or tear in the rectum.

How to Minister:

Tap the cheeks on the face (reflex point) and command the tissues to be healed and fissure to close.

FLU

See Influenza.

FUNGUS

See Infections.

G

GALLSTONES

How to Minister:
1. Lay your hand over the area of the gall bladder, commanding the stones to dissolve.
2. Command the gall bladder to be healed and function normally.

GANGLION CYST

Hard, tumorlike swelling filled with fluid; found usually on the wrist around a tendon or joint.

How to Minister:
1. Lay hands on the affected area, commanding the cyst to dissolve and fluid to reabsorb into the body.
2. Command the wrist structures, bones, muscles, and tendons to go back into normal position.
3. Command the joint lining to produce proper joint fluid and blood supply to be normal.
4. Command all pressure on the nerves to go back to normal.

GLAUCOMA

See Eyes.

GLUTTONY

See chapter 13, "The 'Appestat.'"

GOITER

Swelling of the thyroid gland.

How to Minister:
1. Lay hands on the goiter, and command it to dissolve.
2. Command a new thyroid gland.

GOUT

Deposits of crystals in joints and other organs, usually of the big toe.

How to Minister:
1. Lay hands on the affected foot and command the crystals to dissolve and tissues and bones to be healed.
2. Command the body to metabolize normally.

GUILLIAN-BARRÉ SYNDROME

Nerve deterioration causing paralysis of the body; thought to be caused by viral infection.

How to Minister:
1. Rebuke the infection.
2. Lay hands on the person and command the nervous system to be restored and function perfectly.
3. Command any other structures that have been damaged by the paralysis to become whole.

GUM DISEASE

Diseases of the tissues around the teeth.

How to Minister:
1. Rebuke the infection.
2. Lay hands on the jawbone, commanding the tissues of the mouth to be healed.

H

HAIR LOSS

See Baldness.

HAMMER TOES

See Feet.

HANDS

See Arms and Hands.

Hay Fever
See Allergies.

Headache
Commonly caused by tension, as well as many disease processes (e.g., colds, TMJ, infection, tumors, high blood pressure, etc.).

See Chapter 9, "Migraine Headaches and Tic Douloureux."

How to Minister:
1. Do "TNT," commanding the blood to flow normally and spasms of the vessels to release.
2. Cast out the spirit of migraine (if necessary).
3. Instruct the person to move his head and stretch the neck area. Then ask, "What happened to the pain?"

Heart
Any problem involving the heart.

How to Minister:
1. Speak a new heart into the body.
2. "Grow out the arms" and do "TNT."
3. Command other body parts that have been affected by the heart disease to be healed.

Hemorrhoids
Enlarged blood vessels in the tissues surrounding the rectum.

How to Minister:
1. Tap the person's cheeks (the colon reflex area) and command the hemorrhoids to be healed in Jesus' name.
2. Command the blood vessels to shrink to normal size and function.
3. Rebuke pain.
4. "Grow out the legs" and do "TPT," commanding nerves and muscles to be relaxed and normal.

HEPATITIS C

Hepatitis C makes your liver swell and stops it from working right. You need a healthy liver. The liver does many things to keep you alive. The liver fights infections and stops bleeding. It removes drugs and other poisons from your blood. The liver also stores energy for when you need it.

The Internet has much detail about Hepatitis C.

How to Minister:
1. Command a creative miracle of a new liver. (See Romans 4:17.)
2. In addition to this, command the electrical and chemical frequencies to be in harmony and in balance and to digest the bad cells.

HERNIA

An outpouching of tissue through an area of weakened muscle.

Hiatus Hernia

Protruding of stomach above the diaphragm leading to pain, indigestion, and swallowing difficulties.

How to Minister:
1. "Grow out the arms," commanding all the bones, muscles, nerves, and ligaments to be in proper alignment, strength, and function.
2. Lay hands on the hernia, commanding it to be healed.

Inguinal, Umbilical, or Abdominal Hernia

Outpouching of the intestinal tract in the abdomen, inguinal area (where upper thigh meets the lower abdomen), or umbilicus (belly button).

How to Minister:
1. "Grow out the legs."
2. Do "TPT," commanding the hernia to disappear; muscles, tendons, and tissues to be healed and restored to normal strength.

HERPES

A viral infection affecting various parts of the body.

Herpes Simplex

Commonly called a "cold sore."

Herpes Zoster

Commonly called "shingles."

How to Minister:

1. Command the infection to go.
2. Command the tissues to be healed and restored to normal.

Herpes Simplex (Genital)

"Sores" appear on the external reproductive tissues of the body.
See also Venereal Disease.

HOMOSEXUALS/LESBIANS

Individuals who prefer intimate relationships with others of the same sex; homosexual refers to males, lesbian refers to females. The individual must want to be free from the desire before he can be delivered and healed from this condition.

See chapter 11, "When Ministering Healing."

How to Minister:

1. Lead the person in the prayer of salvation and total commitment. Say, "Father, I will please You and not myself with my lifestyle."
2. Minister the baptism with the Holy Spirit.
3. Bind and cast out the spirit of homosexuality or lesbianism.
4. Command the desires to be heterosexually (desire for the opposite sex) oriented.

HUNTINGTON'S CHOREA

Hereditary disease characterized by involuntary twisting and writhing movements of the extremeties and face, disturbed speech, and impairment of the thoughts.

How to Minister:
1. Cast out the spirits of inheritance and Huntington's disease.
2. Command a new brain to form.

HYPERTENSION (HIGH BLOOD PRESSURE)

Blood pressure that is abnormally high. Ask if cause is known.
See also Fear.

How to Minister:
1. Command a divine "roto-rooter" treatment throughout entire vascular system.
2. Command the blood pressure to return to normal and to remain normal.
3. Suggest time in the Word of God every day and to relax in Jesus, eliminating unnecessary tension, anxiety, and fear.

HYPOGLYCEMIA

Abnormally low blood sugar; sometimes the first indication of early diabetes.

How to Minister:
1. Cast out the spirits of inheritance and hypoglycemia.
2. Command a new pancreas to produce normal blood sugar levels.

I

IMMUNE SYSTEM

See page 161.

How to Minister:

1. Command the immune system to be healed and alert to halt disease and germs from infecting the body in Jesus' name.
2. Command the electrical and chemical frequencies to be in harmony and balance and to digest the sick cells in Jesus' name.

INCURABLE DISEASES

Any disease for which doctors cannot find the cure.
See Chapter 7, "Electrical and Chemical Freequences."

How to Minister:

1. Cast out the spirit of whatever disease is involved.
2. Speak healing to the body.

INFECTION

Caused from numerous organisms (e.g., bacteria, virus, fungus, or parasite).

How to Minister:

1. Rebuke the infection.
2. Command the body to be healed and restored to normal condition and function.
3. Do "TTT."

INFERTILITY

Inability to conceive children.

How to Minister:

1. Say, "Father, Your Word says the womb of Your children shall not be barren, and You will make the barren woman the joyful mother of many children. I speak the first one in here, perfect, whole and delivered within one year."
2. Do "TPT."
3. Command any abnormal formations to become normal.

INFLUENZA, FLU, COLDS

How to Minister:

1. Rebuke the infection.
2. "Grow out the arms" and do "TNT," commanding the blood vessels to open and allow the blood to flow freely to free the affected area(s) of germs.
3. Tell the person to drink eight glasses of water per day to flush germs from system.
4. Command the intestinal symptoms to go in Jesus' name and the body to accept and utilize food normally.

INNER HEALING

Healing of memories (e.g., hurts, insults, cruel treatment) usually caused by another person.

See Chapter 3, "Falling under the Power."

How to Minister:

1. Ask God to take His divine spiritual eraser and remove the hurts of the past.
2. Ask the person to forgive anyone who has hurt him.
3. Lay hands on his head and ask Jesus to bless him. Generally, he will go under the power for the Holy Spirit to minister to him.

INSOMNIA

Inability to sleep.

How to Minister:

1. Speak the peace and love of God into the individual. Recommend that the person spend time in the Word of God and possibly listen to a Bible cassette as he goes to sleep.
2. Command the sleep center of the brain to operate normally.

J

JAW

See TMJ.

JOINTS (FROZEN OR DISLOCATED)

See Chapter 12, "The Spine."

How to Minister:

1. Cast out the spirits of arthritis and bursitis.
2. Do any part of or all of "TTT," as appropriate.
3. Command the joint with its cartilage, ligaments, tendons, and tissues to be healed and loosed as you tap the joint lightly with your hand. Tell the person to begin to move the extremity.
4. If a bone is out of joint, command it to go back into the socket and stay there.

K

KIDNEYS

The organs of the body that remove unnecessary substances from the blood (e.g., fluid, chemicals, etc.) and pass them out of the body in the form of urine.

Kidney Damage or Kidney Failure

Does not pass the excess fluid and/or chemicals out of the body, causing condition that poisons the body; many underlying causes for damage or failure.

How to Minister:

1. Do "TPT" and/or "grow out the legs," commanding a new pair of kidneys to operate and function normally.
2. Command healing for underlying causes (e.g., disease, high blood pressure, infection, etc.).

Kidney Stones

How to Minister:

1. Command the stones to dissolve.
2. Command the pain to go.
3. Command the kidneys and all damaged tissues to be healed and restored to normal function.

202 ⟨♥⟩Handbook for Healing

L

Legs

Kneecap Problems

Can be caused by disease or trauma.

How to Minister:
1. If arthritis, cast out the spirit.
2. Lay hands on the affected area, commanding all the tendons, ligaments, muscles, cartilage and tissues, to be healed; the blood and fluid to lubricate the area to be restored.
3. Command a new kneecap, if needed.
4. "Grow out the legs."

Knock-Knees

How to Minister:
1. Do "TPT," commanding the pelvic bone to rotate outward.
2. "Grow out the legs," commanding the legs and knees to straighten.

Ligaments, Torn or Damaged

Usually caused by twisting or excessive stretching.

How to Minister:
1. Rebuke any infection.
2. "Grow out the arms or legs," as appropriate.
3. Do "TNT" and "TPT," as appropriate.
4. Command the ligaments to be healed and restored to normal function.

Short Leg

Generally caused by a lower back problem that draws up the ligaments, muscles, and bones, making the leg appear to be "short"; leg bone, etc., can actually be permanently shorter because of abnormal development.

How to Minister:
1. "Grow out legs," commanding the back to be healed and muscles and ligaments to go into right position.
2. Do "TPT."
3. If leg is actually shorter or smaller, command a creative miracle—for it to grow to normal length and size.

LEUKEMIA

See Cancer.

LOU GEHRIG'S DISEASE

Also known as Amyotrophic Lateral Sclerosis.

LUMPS

Any abnormal growth in the body.

How to Minister:
1. Curse the core, root, and cause of the lump.
2. Lay hands on the affected area (or on top of the person's hands as he touches the area), commanding the lump to dissolve and disappear.
3. Command all tissues to be healed.

LUNGS (RESPIRATORY RESTRICTIONS)

How to Minister:
Command new lungs, air sacs to open, excess fluid to dry up, or whatever is needed.

LUPUS

Disease when the body attacks itself; can affect many organs in the body including the skin, kidneys, and joints.

How to Minister:
1. Cast out the spirit of lupus.
2. Command the immune system and all affected organs to be healed and to function normally.

M

MACULAR DEGENERATION

See Eyes.

MARRIAGE PROBLEMS

How to Minister:
1. Remind the couple that what they do to each other, they do to Jesus who lives within each of them. Also tell them that their marriage is a practice ground for their marriage to Jesus. Suggest that they go back to the beginning of their love for each other.
2. Ask if they are both saved and Spirit-filled. If not, minister salvation and the baptism with the Spirit to them.
3. Lay hands on each of them—both at the same time (if present)—and speak the peace of God on them. Ask God's blessings on their marriage.
4. If only one is present or saved, ask God to station angels around the unsaved member.

MEASLES

See Infection.

MENIERE'S DISEASE

Disturbance in the inner ear.

Also see Ears.

How to Minister:

1. Cast out the spirit of Meniere's disease.
2. Command the inner ear to be healed, the nerves and blood flow to the inner ear to be normal, and all dizziness to stop.

MENTAL ILLNESS

See Chapter 11, "When Ministering Healing."

How to Minister:

1. Command spirit to come out.
2. If insanity, cast out the insane spirit.
3. If caused by an accident, command a new brain.
4. If a chemical disorder, command the production of proper chemicals in normal amounts.
5. Lay hands for the Holy Spirit to minister to the individual's needs.

MENSTRUAL PAIN

See Female Problems.

MIGRAINE

See Headache.

MONGOLISM

See Down's Syndrome.

MOTION SICKNESS

How to Minister:

1. Command the inner ear to adjust to movements.
2. Lay hands on the head, commanding peace to the brain.

MULTIPLE SCLEROSIS (MS)

See also Chapter 7, "Electrical and Chemical Frequencies."

How to Minister:

1. Bind and cast out the spirit of MS.
2. Do "TTT," commanding the nerves to be healed and restored to normal structure and function.
3. Command healing and normal function to all parts of the body that have been affected by the disease.

MUSCULAR DYSTROPHY (MD)

Progressive degeneration of muscles.

See also Chapter 7, "Electrical and Chemical Frequencies."

How to Minister:

1. Cast out the spirit of muscular dystrophy.
2. Do "TTT," commanding the muscles to be healed, restored, and to function normally.

MYASTHENIA GRAVIS

Disease characterized by weakness and rapid tiring of voluntary skeletal muscles.

How to Minister:

1. Cast out the spirit of myasthenia gravis.
2. Do "TTT," commanding the nerve receptors on the muscles to be healed and function normally.

N

NARCOLEPSY

Uncontrollable episodes of sleep during normal waking hours.

How to Minister:

1. Cast out the spirit of narcolepsy.
2. Lay hands on the head, commanding the sleep center of the brain to be healed and to function normally.

NECK

Including muscle strain, pain, and/or cracked vertebrae.

How to Minister:
1. Do "TNT."
2. Command vertebrae, discs, muscles, ligaments, nerves, and tendons to be healed and to go back into normal position.

NERVOUSNESS

See also Fear, Anxiety.

How to Minister:
1. Cast out the spirits of fear and anxiety.
2. Lay hands on the person's head and speak the peace of God into the mind.

NOSE

Deformed or broken.

How to Minister:
Lay your finger on the nose and run it down the crest, commanding it to be straight, structures to be regenerated, and to function normally.

NUMBNESS

Caused by disease or pinching of the nerves.

How to Minister:
1. Command any disease process to go.
2. Do "TTT," commanding discs and vertebrae of the back to return to normal position, pressure on the nerves to be released, and nerves to function normally.

O

OBESITY

Condition of being excessively overweight.
See Chapter 13, "The Appestat."

How to Minister:

Lay hands on the head and command the "appestat" (appetite control center) to be readjusted to the normal level and weight to return to correct and healthy range.

OSTEOARTHRITIS

See Arthritis.

OSTEOPOROSIS (DOWAGER'S HUMP)

Deterioration of bones.

How to Minister:

1. Cast out the spirit of osteoporosis.
2. Do "TTT," commanding the bones to use the calcium and other necessary minerals in the body to regenerate new, strong bones.
3. Command the back and sacrum to straighten.

P

PALSY

See Parkinson's Disease.

PARKINSON'S DISEASE

Degeneration of cells in the base of the brain accompanied by shaking.
See Chapter 7, "Electrical and Chemical Frequencies."

How to Minister:

1. Cast out the spirit of Parkinson's disease.
2. Do "TNT," commanding a new brain and nerve tissue that will function normally.
3. Command healing to all other affected parts of the body.

PHLEBITIS
Irritation of blood vessels.

How to Minister:
1. Command blood clot to dissolve.
2. Command infection to leave.

PITUITARY GLAND
Endocrine gland located at base of the brain.
See Chapter 13, "The Appestat."

How to Minister:
1. If cause is known, minister to cause.
2. Lay hands on the person's head and/or do "TNT," commanding the pituitary gland to function properly and produce normal amounts of all its hormones.
3. Command all other affected body parts to become normal.

POLIO, POLIOMYELITIS
Infectious virus.
See Chapter 7, "Electrical and Chemical Frequencies."

How to Minister:
1. Cast out the spirit of polio.
2. Do "TTT," commanding creative miracles to the spinal cord and its damaged nerves, muscles, ligaments, tissues, and tendons to be healed, strengthen, and function normally.

PMS (PREMENSTRUAL SYNDROME)
See Female Problems.

PREGNANCY
See Birth, Infertility.

PROLAPSED UTERUS
See Female Problems.

PROSTATE TROUBLE

Enlargement of male reproductive gland.
See Chapter 7, "Electrical and Chemical Frequencies."

How to Minister:

1. "Grow out the legs" and do "TPT," commanding the prostate gland to shrink to normal size and to function normally.
2. Command nerves and blood to work normally.

PSORIASIS

Skin disease.

How to Minister:

1. Cast out the spirit of psoriasis.
2. Rebuke the inflammation, itching, and scaling.
3. Lay hands near (not on) the affected areas, commanding healthy new skin cells to replace the affected tissues.

R

RESPIRATORY DISEASE

See Lungs.

RETARDATION

Inability to develop or learn normally; may be caused by brain damage or disease.

How to Minister:

1. Cast out spirit of inheritance.
2. Lay hands on the head, commanding a new brain with normal intelligence.

RETINITIS PIGMENTOSA

See Eyes.

RHEUMATIC FEVER

How to Minister:
1. Rebuke the infection.
2. Do "TTT," commanding the joints, heart, and other tissues of the body to be healed and react normally.
3. Command any damaged organs to be healed and function properly.

RHEUMATOID ARTHRITIS

See Arthritis.

How to Minister:
In addition to the ministering mentioned under Arthritis, command the immune system to be healed.

RINGING IN THE EARS

See Ears.

S

SCARS, KELOIDS, ADHESIONS

Keloids: abnormal scars on skin.

Adhesions: abnormal growing together of tissues and/or organs inside the body; usually following surgery.

How to Minister:
1. Do whichever of "TTT" that relates to the affected area, commanding the scar tissue to be dissolved.
2. Command all organs and structures to be healed and to function normally.

SCHIZOPHRENIA

See Mental Illness.

212 ❤️ *Handbook for Healing*

SCIATICA

Pain running along large nerves from spine into thigh.

How to Minister:

1. "Grow out the legs" and do "TPT," commanding the lumbar vertebra and sacrum to be properly aligned.
2. Command all the discs to go back into place and relieve all pressure on the nerves.
3. Place your fingers on either side of the spine above the sacrum and command the sciatica spirit to come out.

SCLERODERMA

Skin feels like it is turning to stone.

How to Minister:

1. Cast out the spirit of scleroderma.
2. Do "TTT," commanding the immune system to be healed and return to normal function.
3. Command new tissue to replace the damaged areas of the skin and all affected internal organs.

SCOLIOSIS

Abnormal curvature of the spine.

How to Minister:

1. Cast out the spirit of scoliosis.
2. Do "TTT," commanding the bones in the back, the ribs, and supportive structures of the body to come into alignment.

SICKLE-CELL ANEMIA

Hereditary disease; red blood cells become "sickle" shaped and clog blood vessels.

How to Minister:

1. Cast out the spirit of inheritance.
2. Command the defective genes to be restored to normal and marrow to produce normal blood cells, and the affected organs and tissues of the body to be healed.

SINUS PROBLEMS

How to Minister:
1. Rebuke the infection and curse the allergy.
2. Lay hands on the face and command the sinuses to drain, open up, and be healed.
3. "Grow out the arms," commanding blood vessels to open and reduce swelling of the areas.
4. Suggest that the person avoid irritating factors (sugar, caffeine, and nicotine aggravate sinus infection).
5. Drinking eight glasses of water (and juice) daily will alleviate the problem also.

SPINA BIFIDA

Birth defect in the spine.

How to Minister:
Speak a creative miracle into the body. Command spine to close.

STOMACH

Also see Ulcers.

How to Minister:
1. Determine specific defect and command it to be healed or new part created.
2. Do "TPT" and "grow out the legs."

STROKE

Blockage of a blood vessel leading to the brain.

How to Minister:
1. Cast out the spirit of death of brain cells.
2. Lay hands on the head, commanding the blockage to dissolve and be removed; all damaged tissue be restored; a creative miracle—a new brain, if necessary.
3. Do "TTT," commanding the communication from the brain to the body and all affected parts of the body be restored to normal function.
4. See details in *How to Heal the Sick.*

SUICIDE

Taking your own life.
See Chapter 11, "When Ministering Healing."

How to Minister:

1. Bind and cast out the spirit of suicide.
2. Lead the person in the prayer of salvation and minister the baptism with the Holy Spirit.
3. Urge the individual to attend a good church with a Spirit-filled pastor. If possible, make this connection for him.
4. Recommend that he spend a lot of time reading a modern version of the Bible, and other good books, such as *Let This Mind Be in You* by Frances.

T

TAILBONE (COCCYX)

Lowest bone of the spinal column.

How to Minister:

1. Cast out the spirit of death of brain cells.
2. Lay hands on the head, commanding the blockage to dissolve and be removed; all damaged tissue be restored; a creative miracle—a new brain, if necessary.
3. Do "TTT," commanding the communication from the brain to the body and all affected parts of the body be restored to normal function.
4. See details in *How to Heal the Sick.*

TEETH

Crooked

How to Minister:

1. Cast out the spirit of inheritance.
2. Lay hands on the jaw, commanding the jaws to be adjusted to allow enough space for the teeth to be in proper alignment.
3. Command the teeth to line up properly.

Decay

How to Minister:
1. Curse the decay.
2. Lay hands on the jaw, commanding a creative miracle— teeth to be restored and covered with a perfect layer of enamel.

Grinding

Usually occurs at night while asleep. See also TMJ.

How to Minister:
1. Do "TNT" and "grow out the arms," commanding nerves to be released.
2. Speak the mind of Christ into the person and suggest that he spend time in the Bible.
3. If necessary, deal with unforgiveness.

Overbite or Underbite

Caused by jaw being out of place.
See also TMJ.

How to Minister:
1. Cast out the spirit of inheritance.
2. Lay hands on the jaw, commanding the jaw to be adjusted to allow enough space for the teeth to be in proper alignment.
3. Command the teeth to line up properly.

TMJ SYNDROME

Inflammation of the "hinge-joint" of the jaw.

How to Minister:
1. Do "TTT," commanding the jaw to go back into place.
2. Command the tissues, ligaments, and cartilage to be healed and adjusted to the right alignment.

TENDONITIS

Inflammation and/or irritation of the tendons.

How to Minister:
1. Rebuke the inflammation.
2. Do the appropriate portion of "TTT" (e.g., "grow out the arms" for the elbow and shoulder, "grow out the legs" for the knee or hip), commanding the tendon and its surrounding tissues to be healed.
3. Command the pain, all swelling, and irritation to go.

THYROID DISEASE

How to Minister:
1. Do "TNT."
2. Speak a creative miracle—a new thyroid gland.

TIC DOULOUREUX

Severe pain in the side of the face.
See Chapter 9, "Migraine Headaches and Tic Douloureux."

How to Minister:
Do "TNT," commanding the pain to go and the nerve to be healed.

TINNITUS

See Ears.

TONSILITIS

How to Minister:
1. Rebuke the infection.
2. Do "TNT," commanding the tonsils to shrink to normal size and to function normally.

TWITCHING

How to Minister:

Lay hands on the affected area, commanding all pressure to be relieved, all irritation be gone, and the nerves to be healed.

U

ULCERS

Open sores in the stomach or small intestine; can also be on skin.

How to Minister:

1. Command tissues in the affected area to be healed—a new lining, if necessary.
2. Do "TTT," commanding the stomach to produce acid in normal levels.
3. Speak the peace of God into the person's mind and heart.

UTERUS

See Female Problems.

V

VARICOSE VEINS

Veins (usually of the legs) that have become abnormally dilated.

How to Minister:

1. Cast out the spirit of inheritance.
2. "Grow out the legs," commanding the vessel walls to strengthen and function normally, any blockage to be removed, and the blood to flow normally back to the heart.

VENEREAL DISEASE

Disease passed through sexual relations. Includes gonorrhea, syphillis, AIDS, some forms of herpes.

How to Minister:
1. If the disease was passed during a sinful act, be sure the person has repented and promised God he or she would not repeat the sexual sin again.
2. Minister salvation and the baptism with the Spirit.
3. Rebuke the infection.
4. Cast out the spirit of lust, if appropriate.
5. Lay hands on the person, commanding healing to all affected body parts, creative miracles as necessary, and the blood to be clean and clear.
6. Command the immune system to be restored to normal for those with AIDS.

VERTIGO

See Ears.

W

WARTS

How to Minister:
1. Curse the seed and the root of the wart.
2. Command the wart to dry up and fall off.
3. Tell the person to say, "Thank You, Jesus," until the warts fall off.

WATER ON THE KNEE OR ELBOW

See Edema.

WEIGHT LOSS

How to Minister:

1. Ask what the doctor considers to be the cause.
2. Minister to the cause.
3. Command the "appestat" to be readjusted to normal and the body to adjust to a proper weight.

WHIPLASH

Usually the result of a car accident.

How to Minister:

1. Do "TTT."
2. Command any damaged disc, vertebrae, nerve, ligament, tendon, or muscle to be healed.

Z

ZZZ

Lack of insomnia.

Books by Charles and Frances Hunter

The Angel Book[†]
Born Again! What Do You Mean?
A Confession a Day Keeps the Devil Away
Don't Be Afraid of Fear[*]
Follow Me
God Is Fabulous
God's Answer to Fat—Loose It!
God's Big "IF"[*]
God's Healing Promises[†]
Heealing Through Humor
Hotline to Heaven
How Do You Treat My Son, Jesus?
How to Develop Your Faith[*]

How to Heal the Sick†
How to Make the Word Come Alive
How to Make Your Marriage Exciting
How to Pick a Perfect Husband...or Wife
How to Receive and Maintain a Healing
How to Receive and Minister the Baptism
*with the Holy Spirit**
Impossible Miracles
Let This Mind Be in You†
*Memorizing Made Easy**
*Shout the Word—Stop the Thief**
Skinnie Minnie Recipe Book
Strength for Today
Supernatural Horizons
*There Are Two Kinds Of...**
The Two Sides of a Coin
*What's in a Name?**

*Indicates a mini-book.
†Indicates a book published by Whitaker House,
New Kensington, PA 15068.

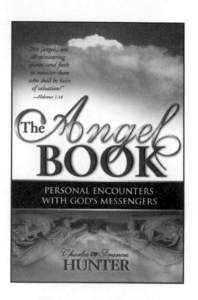

The Angel Book:
Personal Encounters with God's Messengers
Charles and Frances Hunter

Charles and Frances Hunter describe their own personal encounters with angels and what the Bible tells us about these messengers of God. They report on the different kinds of angels and their roles, how God's messengers can impact your life, and how to experience the presence of God. Discover how God uses angels to bring answers to prayer, to wage spiritual warfare, to communicate His will to us, and to strengthen us during trials.

ISBN: 0-88368-598-1 • Trade • 224 pages

WHITAKER
HOUSE

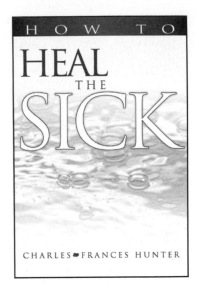

How to Heal the Sick

Charles and Frances Hunter

A loved one is sick, your friend was just in an accident,
a family member is facing an emotional crisis. Have you
ever desperately longed to reach out your hand and bring
healing to your loved ones? At times our hearts ache
with the desire to help. What you, as a Christian, need to
know is that the Holy Spirit within you is ready to heal the
sick! The Hunters present solid, biblically-based methods
of healing that can bring you physical health, spiritual
wholeness, and abundant life.

ISBN: 0-88368-600-7 • Trade • 224 pages

**WHITAKER
HOUSE**

proclaiming the power of the Gospel through the written word
visit our website at www.whitakerhouse.com

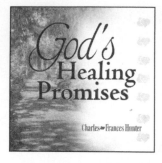

There is healing in God's words, because they are words of promise. Here are God's life-giving words, interspersed with faith-affirming testimonies, to bring you health and restoration. Saturate yourself in these expressions of healing, apply them to yourself, and receive the promise of His Word.

God's Healing Promises
Charles and Frances Hunter
ISBN: 0-88368-630-9 • 6" x 6" Gift Book • 176 pages

I Promise...Love, God
Charles and Frances Hunter
ISBN: 0-88368-668-6 • 7" x 8" Gift Book • 336 pages

God is sending you a message—a message of His love for you. Have you been ignoring His efforts? He wants to tell you about all His promises. He wants you to understand that the promises in His Word are true and that they're for you. Now that God has your attention and can give you directions, you can be on the road to an exciting, joy-filled life!

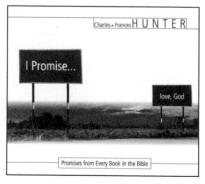

ШJ
WHITAKER
HOUSE

proclaiming the power of the Gospel through the written word
visit our website at www.whitakerhouse.com